To our colleagues – students, mentors, teachers and researchers.
Thanks for giving it a go.

Reflective Practice in Nursing

4th Edition

Edited by

Chris Bulman
RGN, RNT, MSc, BSc (Hons), PGCEA
Formerly Senior Lecturer, School of Health and
Social Care, Oxford Brookes University
Part-time PhD student, University of Southampton

Sue Schutz
MSc, RGN, Cert Ed (FE)
Senior Lecturer, School of Health and Social Care,
Oxford Brookes University
Part-time MPhil/PhD student,
University of Southampton

Blackwell
Publishing

Library of Congress Cataloging-in-Publication Data

Reflective practice in nursing / edited by Chris Bulman and Sue Schutz. – 4th ed.
p. ; cm.
Includes bibliographical references and index.
ISBN-13: 978-1-4051-7360-5 (pbk. : alk. paper)
1. Nursing–Philosophy. 2. Critical thinking
I. Bulman, Chris. II. Schutz, Sue.
[DNLM: 1. Nursing. 2. Education, Nursing. 3. Learning. 4. Nursing Process. 5. Philosophy, Nursing. 6. Thinking. WY 16 R332 2008]

RT84.5.R455 2008
610.7301–dc22
2008002536

A catalogue record for this book is available from the British Library.

Set in 10/12 pt Avenir by SNP Best-set Typesetter Ltd., Hong Kong
Printed in Great Britain by TJ International Ltd, Padstow, Cornwall

3 2011

Contents

Contributors

Editors

Chris Bulman   RGN, RNT, MSc, BSc (Hons), PGCEA, Formerly Senior Lecturer, School of Health and Social Care, Oxford Brookes University.

Sue Schutz   MSc, RGN, Cert Ed (FE), Senior Lecturer, School of Health and Social Care, Oxford Brookes University.

Contributors

Jane M. Appleton   RGN, BA (Hons), MSc, PGDE, Quality and Learning Manager, Sue Ryder Care.

Sue Atkins   MSc, RN, RM, Dip N, Dip N Ed, Principal Lecturer, School of Health and Social Care, Oxford Brookes University.

Bernie Carter   PhD, PGCE, BSc, RSCN, SRN, Professor of Children's Nursing, Families, Children and Life Transitions Research Group, Department of Nursing, University of Central Lancashire.

Sue Duke   PhD, MSc, BSc, PGDE, RN, RNT, Consultant Practitioner in Cancer and Palliative Care/Senior Lecturer, School of Nursing and Midwifery, University of Southampton.

Melanie Jasper   PhD, MSc, BNurs, BA, RGN, RM, RHV, NDNCert, PGCEA, MILT, Professor and Head of School of Health Science Glyndwr Building, University of Swansea.

Charlotte Maddison   MSc, BA (Hons), RGN, Senior Lecturer, School of Health and Social Care, Oxford Brookes University.

Pam Sharp   MSc, PG Dip, RGN, Senior Lecturer, School of Health and Social Care, Oxford Brookes University.

Elizabeth Walker   BA, RGN, RCNT, DPNS, RM, Formerly Senior Lecturer, Division of Adult Post-Registration Nursing, Department of Nursing, University of Central Lancashire.

Preface

Welcome to the fourth edition of *Reflective Practice in Nursing*. This new edition responds to the continued interest in reflective practice amongst nurses and offers a motivating and accessible text about reflection. Fundamentally this book does not assume any previous knowledge about reflection and aims to be of practical use to those wanting to learn about reflection and what it may have to offer them.

Past editions of *Reflective Practice in Nursing* have been read by a wide variety of nurses; from pre- and post-registration students, and from diploma to master's level. It has had appeal for practitioners from a huge range of backgrounds and experience, as well as teachers, managers, mentors and professionals from other disciplines. The success of these other editions has motivated us to continue to communicate our experience and our growing knowledge in using reflection.

We hope the fourth edition has much new to offer. The updated first chapter introduces you to reflection and considers some philosophical underpinnings. It looks at why nurses might be interested in reflection and presents theory and research from the disciplines of nursing and education. This chapter is useful if you are new to reflection and also for re-examining your thinking, even if you have some experience of it already. Chapter 2 on skills for reflection has also been updated to include an appreciation of attributes for reflection as well as issues to do with influencing change as a reflective practitioner.

Chapter 3 on assessing and evaluating reflection remains and has been extensively added to and updated. This is a challenging area for debate but remains one that we feel needs to continue to be raised, if practice knowledge is to be valued on an equal footing with theoretical knowledge. We have also amalgamated work on the student's and the mentor's journey with the process of reflection; Chapter 4 focuses on pre-registration students in particular. A revised chapter on writing journals for learning (Chapter 7) and a new chapter on group reflection (Chapter 6) also offer plenty of advice and tips for practitioners and educationalists, as well as a lively critique of the literature.

We continue to be committed to presenting insights into the reality of reflection for those involved in teaching and learning about it. Thus a new chapter is included which details the development of reflection within a post-registration nursing programme (Chapter 5). We believe this work will be particularly valuable to educationalists and all those who support others developing reflection. Additionally, there is much inspiration in Chapter 8 which continues to explore our intrepid practitioner's journey with reflection as she/he progresses with her/his career. Finally, Chapter 9 gives an extensively revised guide to 'having a go' at reflection, drawing on other areas of the book and giving more hints, tips and cautions for getting started with some reflections of your own.

This new edition also tries to convey something of the spirit of the times, which is proving challenging for the education of health care professionals and in the UK is particularly marked by cutbacks in staff, which have a profound effect on the preparation and continuing education of nurses.

Finally, reflection is not without its critics; indeed we hope that we have managed to convey some of the problematic issues as well as the positive aspects. Healthy debate and critical discussion are important and we hope you get a sense of this as you compare and contrast the views of different authors. In essence, our aim is to make you curious about reflection, in a way that gets you thinking about the issues involved and challenges you to look at your view of the world. Essentially we hope it will be useful to all those involved and interested in developing, using and investigating reflective practice.

Chapter 1
An introduction to reflection
Chris Bulman

Introduction

The first edition of this book was published in 1994 and whilst times have certainly changed since then, reflection continues to be of interest to nurses and to influence nursing education around the world. It is a concept that myself and fellow authors remain committed to; hence the development of this book, documenting our experiences, exploring the debates, reviewing the research and offering advice on reflection and reflective education.

We hope the book will help you to make up your own mind about reflection, because we have critiqued some of the issues and put forward some theoretical background in order to help you get a grasp of what reflection is. It is, as always, wise to use your own informed judgement when considering reflection, otherwise, as FitzGerald and Chapman (2000) caution, one prevalent discourse simply replaces another and the ideas associated with that dominant discourse become so influential that alternative views, especially minority views, are in danger of being marginalised. Prudent words aside, in publishing this book we are in effect 'declaring our hand' in that we obviously believe there are benefits to be gained from using reflection. However, we are aware of the difficulties and criticisms, which any good academic and practical debate should not ignore.

What is reflection?

Getting to grips with the concept of reflection is a useful starting point, so long as you bear in mind Chris Johns' (2000) warning against accepting definitions at face value and his comment that practitioners may grasp at theoretical definitions and then struggle to fit the experiences to the definition rather than using the definition to creatively guide reflection. In fact, reflection is a difficult concept to define (James and Clarke 1994;

Clarke *et al.* 1996), and consequently it is interpreted in the literature in slightly different ways.

I see reflection as reviewing experience from practice so that it may be described, analysed, evaluated and consequently used to inform and change future practice. Importantly, reflection also involves opening up one's practice for others to examine, and consequently requires courage and open-mindedness as well as a willingness to take on board and act on criticism (Dewey 1933). In this context, reflection involves more than 'intellectual thinking' since it is intermingled with practitioners' feelings and emotions and acknowledges an interrelationship with action. My views are based on my experiences in using and researching reflection and also from my exploration of the literature, some of which is presented below. As you read through other people's definitions you should begin to see how my views have been influenced by their writing and consequently start to form your own judgements about what the concept of reflection means to you.

I begin with the educationalist and philosopher John Dewey simply because his writing has been so influential in subsequent discussion about the concept. Dewey developed his ideas on thinking and learning and focused on the concept of thinking reflectively. He defined reflection as:

> 'Active, persistent and careful consideration of any belief or supposed form of knowledge in the light of the grounds that support it and the further conclusions to which it tends.' (Dewey 1933, p.9)

Dewey saw reflective thinking as *thinking with a purpose* and focused strongly on the need to test out and challenge true beliefs by applying the scientific method through deductive reasoning and experimentation. He implied that emotions and feelings are part of reflective thinking, but, interestingly, this is not something that he expanded on. He made some important assumptions about people, emphasising our tendencies towards quick solutions, tradition and 'mental ruts' and the pervading influence of culture and the environment upon our thinking. He also emphasised the need for thinking to be directly linked with action, demonstrating the pragmatic nature of his philosophy, and suggested that any thinking can be intellectual, thus emphasising the importance of the practical as well as the theoretical. His philosophy has had a major influence on educational ideas and has certainly influenced the work of Boyd and Fales (1983), Schön (1983, 1987) and Boud *et al.* (1985).

The philosopher Donald Schön has also been a great influence on the development of reflection in professional education and his work inspired the development of reflective education at Oxford Polytechnic, now Oxford Brookes University (Champion 1992; George 1986, unpublished observations). Schön defines reflection-on-action as:

'Thinking back on what we have done in order to discover how our knowing in action may have contributed to an unexpected outcome. We may do so after the fact, in tranquillity or we may pause in the midst of action (stop and think).' (1987, p.26)

His concept of reflection-on-action focuses on retrospective critical thinking, to construct and re-construct events in order to develop oneself as a practitioner and person. Importantly reflection-on-action involves more than 'intellectual' thinking because it is intermingled with the practitioner's feelings and emotions and acknowledges an interrelationship with action (Dewey 1933; Schön 1983, 1987, 1992).

Schön also defines reflection-in-action as happening:

'Where we may reflect in the midst of action without interrupting it. Our thinking serves to reshape what we are doing while we are doing it.' (1987, p.26)

As you can see, this is a different concept from reflection-on-action since it is not about carrying out a 'post mortem' (however speedy) on an experience but concerns thinking and knowing in the midst of action. Schön saw reflection-in-action as a distinguishing feature of expert practitioners who are able to experiment and think about their practice whilst they are doing it; this idea is fundamental to his theory of professional expertise. This is difficult to conceptualise and you will find it is sometimes misrepresented by those who view reflection-on-action and reflection-in-action as the same, and there are authors who critique the whole concept of reflection-in-action (Eraut 1994; Clinton 1998). In this book our main concerns are with the construction of rational and affective knowledge in order to make a positive difference to practice and thus you will find that what authors within these pages are mainly talking about is reflection-on-action.

Nurses have also attempted to offer a definition of reflection based on their interpretation of other theorists and on their own experiences. Whilst working as a practitioner, Brigid Reid formulated this definition after reviewing the work of Boyd and Fales (1983) and Boud et al. (1985), in order to develop a working definition that captured theoretical interpretation and could also be usefully used to teach and facilitate nurses' learning about reflection for the first time.

'Reflection is a process of reviewing an experience of practice in order to describe, analyse, evaluate and so inform learning about practice.' (Reid 1993, p.306)

The educationalists that inspired Brigid Reid to formulate her definition of reflection were themselves influenced by philosophical critical enquiry stemming from the work of Habermas and other members of the

Frankfurt School. Thus the influence of critical theory can be seen in these and other definitions of reflection. As concisely described by Mulhall and Le May (1999, p.120), this is the theory that society is structured by meanings, rules and habits which we adhere to. Its purpose is to unmask those aspects of society that restrict/limit human freedom and maintain the status quo. The central contention of the theory is that each of us is located historically and socially, and as a consequence objective knowledge is dismissed. Thus the importance of emancipatory learning which challenges the status quo was apparent within these definitions:

> 'Reflective learning is the process of internally examining and exploring an issue of concern, triggered by an experience, which creates and clarifies meaning in terms of self and which results in a changed conceptual perspective.' (Boyd and Fales 1983, p.113)

> 'Reflection in the context of learning is a generic term for those intellectual and affective activities in which individuals engage to explore their experiences in order to lead to new understandings and appreciations.' (Boud et al. 1985, p.19)

Saylor (1990, p.8) is another nurse who developed a definition of reflection. She was influenced by the work of Schön, additionally drawing on her own experience as a nurse teacher:

> 'Reflection is a process of reviewing one's repertoire of clinical experience and knowledge to invent novel approaches to complex clinical problems. Reflection also provides data for self evaluation and increases learning from experience.'

Furthermore Clarke and Graham (1996, p.26) defined the process of reflection as follows:

> 'By engaging in reflection people are usually engaging in a period of thinking in order to examine often complex experiences or situations. The period of thinking (reflection) allows the individual to make sense of an experience, perhaps to liken the experience to other similar experiences and to place it in context. Faced with complex decisions thinking it through (reflecting) allows the individual to separate out the various influencing factors and come to a reasoned decision or course of action.'

Wong et al. (1997) described the central point of reflection as experience, with the trigger point of the process usually starting with an emotional response (Dewey 1933), which can be both positive (Boud et al.1985) and uncomfortable (Atkins and Murphy 1993). Like Clarke and Graham they described the reflective process as one of making sense of an experience and learning from it.

These definitions and descriptions demonstrate only some of what is offered in the literature. I have presented those that represent influential philosophical and educational thinkers. Moreover, since this is a book on reflective practice in nursing, I have also considered interpretations of the concept by nurses. Essentially these definitions accentuate that there is no universal definition of reflection in the literature. The reality is that some things are hard to define and so a unanimously agreed definition for reflection may not be a possibility. It seems to me then that we need to pay more attention to how we as nurses identify the meaning of reflection within our practice and thus what similarities and differences we recognise in our interpretations (Wittgenstein 1967).

If you look carefully at the definitions that are presented here, you will certainly begin to notice some similarities; for instance the exploration of experience, the analysis of feelings and of oneself to inform learning. You will also see elements of critical theory where there is an assumption that reflection will involve a changed perspective and action. It is also possible to see elements of experimentation and review and learning through one's experience. There are inevitably differences too; not all emphasise the significance of feelings and emotion, or explicitly recognise the inclusion of change, for instance. Additionally some do not overtly mention the importance of having a sounding board or coach with whom to reflect, suggesting a more solitary interpretation of reflection. In essence, it seems to me that it is necessary to do some reading for yourself, as well as taking a look at how you operate in practice, to begin to consider what you make of reflection.

Why are nurses interested in reflection?

Like other professional groups, nursing has only recently moved into higher education and this has not been without its tensions (Jarvis 1983; Eraut 1994). For nursing this has meant existing within an educational system that historically promotes the division of theoretical and practical knowledge and which traditionally denies an interrelationship between intellect and emotion (Barnett 1992; Reed and Ground 1997; Brockbank and McGill 1998). This philosophical legacy promoted the idea that intellectual knowledge is different from and is superior to practical knowledge and originated from the early philosophers such as Plato (Day 1994), but was strongly influenced by later Cartesian theory which viewed the mind as something separate from the body. Descartes' propositions promoted the concept of dualism, advocating thinking skills as separate from feelings and from action (Cottingham 1997). Other philosophers began to appreciate thinking from an inherently different stance, arguing that the mind and body are interconnected and that knowledge is socially rather than individually constructed and thus that thinking, feelings and action are intertwined (Ryle 1963, 1979; Wittgenstein 1967; Bloor 1983; Canfield 1986; Hacker 1997).

Eraut (1994) warned of the tensions between such university and professionally orientated perspectives on knowledge. Universities seek to develop and broaden academic knowledge and consequently to challenge long-established professional practices. He also discussed the difficulties with integrating professional education into higher education, citing the difference between propositional knowledge, i.e. that pertaining to or of the nature of a logical proposition (New Shorter Oxford English Dictionary 1993) and 'know how'. This is a point amply illustrated by the philosophers cited above under the assumption that propositional knowledge is the most 'truthful' form of knowledge. This exposes the influence of western philosophy on the importance and status of propositional knowledge in society and raises again the problem of dualism in the valuing of knowledge.

In a similar vein, Polanyi's (1958, 1967) influential work offered a critique of the ideal of objectivity as it was presented in science and philosophy in the mid-twentieth century. He suggested that complete objectivity as attributed to science is a delusion and a false ideal. In this way, Polanyi pointed out the requirement to look at how personal knowing influences and enhances the objective. He also suggested a need to appreciate the knowledge that is embodied through practical knowing, e.g. the nurse develops a 'feel' for what she does practically and bodily so that it becomes part of her knowing process. However, this kind of knowledge cannot always be articulated in words; as Polanyi suggested, 'we know more than we can say'. Consequently he advised of the need to provide adequate ways to help people to express themselves, and reflection has the potential for providing such a means. Polanyi's work suggests that our tacit knowing will never be expressed, yet reflection potentially offers a key to unlocking the expression of some things that previously we were not able to communicate. This is because, with the right support as well as challenge, reflection has the potential to ease the way for and open up dialogue and also to provide a language with which to express our practice to others.

Why change to reflection?

Nursing is a practice discipline, and effective preparation of nurses requires that we are able to care competently for clients and continue to develop skills and knowledge over a professional lifetime. This means learning certain skills and particular knowledge, and developing attitudes and attributes that allow us to nurse in an effective and sensitive way that makes a positive difference to our clients (Paterson and Zderad 1988; McMahon and Pearson 1998). A traditional way of achieving this is through what Schön (1983, 1987) called *technical rationality*, where students learn about theory and then apply this to their practice, echoing the separation of intellectual and practical knowledge that I have outlined above. No doubt many of you will be able to identify this style of education when you look back at some of your own experiences.

The interest in reflection is timely in relation to the climate of change in higher education more generally. The 'banking' notion of education, where students were 'filled up' with knowledge, as described by Freire (1972), is being challenged by a greater emphasis on and interest in enabling students to learn how to learn through the development of effective critical thinking skills (Brookfield 1987; Gibbs *et al.* 1988; Barnett 1992; Jarvis *et al.* 2003). Additionally there is interesting educational work that advocates the importance and effectiveness of learning through experience (Rogers 1983; Boud *et al.* 1985; Gibbs *et al.* 1988; Clift *et al.* 1990; Jarvis *et al.* 2003). There has also been specific criticism of the technical rational approach to professional education, characterised by students learning about theory and attempting to apply it to practice (Schön 1983, 1987; Eraut 1994). This fails to recognise the need to bridge the so-called theory–practice gap, to educate nurses to learn from their practice, develop their thinking and ultimately make a difference to their clients' care.

Freire's (1972) notion of praxis or action that is informed and linked to certain values is influential to my beliefs about reflection. It is this notion of praxis that emphasises the requirement to make a positive difference to clients, to avoid 'automatic pilot' and strive to develop responsive, purposeful and understanding practice. This is necessary because of the commitment to do the best that we can for those that are in need of nursing. Freire's notion of praxis and the belief of its central place in any contemplation about reflection also resonates with Barnett's (1997) notion of *critical being*. Principally, Barnett challenged the idea of critical thinking as it has developed and is traditionally supported within higher education. He advocated the nurturing of critical being in students rather than critical thinking. By its very nature, critical being encapsulates the development of critical thinking but also the critical development of self and the commitment to take action in the world. Although Barnett was chiefly deconstructing traditional notions of critical thinking (he did critique reflective practice and professionals in his work and this is also worth a read), it is the essence of his work on critical being that resonates with my thoughts on the nature of reflection. We should not discard the use of propositional knowledge in reflection or become distracted by its status but rather say that reflection becomes an intermingling of different sorts of knowing that should include feelings, self awareness and a commitment to action.

✳ In summary, nurses are interested in reflection because it provides a vehicle through which they can communicate and justify the importance of practice and practice knowledge. This in effect begins to legitimise knowledge derived from the realities of practice rather than simply from more traditional forms of knowing (Brockbank and McGill 1998). Consequently, nursing education has begun to integrate reflection into the preparation and continuing professional development of nurses. Such influences can be specifically identified in United Kingdom Central Council for Nursing, Midwifery and Health Visiting (UKCC) documents dating from the mid-1990s (UKCC 1994, 1996) and in Nursing and Midwifery Council (NMC) publications (NMC 2004a–c, 2005).

What does reflection have to offer nurses?

So far I have conveyed the lack of recognition of personal and practice knowledge in higher education generally and the consequent issues for nurse education. This is in accordance with philosophical propositions about the nature of knowing and thinking where thinking, feelings and action are intermingled (Ryle 1963; Wittgenstein 1967). It is important for nurses to find a way to communicate their stories and feelings about practice in ways that cannot be achieved through a traditional technical route, or can be found in conventional nursing textbooks. The value of acknowledging and learning from this type of thinking and knowing is powerfully captured by Sue Duke (2000):

> 'Nursed a patient tired of fighting, feeling hopeless. I stayed with the patient but my heart emptied of anything that could protect me.' (Duke 2000, p.138)

Sue Duke wrote this extract as a reflective diary entry. Taking time later to look back on it, she described being stunned by how she had managed to capture her feelings about caring for a person. She started to wonder how many times before she had felt like that and had simply forgotten how she felt and why. For her this began a long process of attending to, and reflectively writing about, her practice, providing her with an opportunity to learn from it. Sue's journey is continued in Chapter 8 of this book.

Significantly, current thinking in nursing advocates the need for nurses to be educated in ways that develop their autonomy, critical thinking, ability to be sensitive to others and open-mindedness (Reed and Ground 1997). This reflects the demands and expectations made on nurses and the health services that they work within. Duke's example above illustrates the opportunity to liberate and use every-day practice experience for learning and thus the potential for reflection to develop oneself and one's practice.

What sort of information is there in the literature regarding reflection?

The world-wide interest in reflection has accordingly generated an enormous amount of literature on the subject. Within the confines of this chapter I have put together a résumé of nursing research, discussion and clinical papers. Numerous others are discussed throughout other chapters in the book. The discussion papers and what I have called clinical papers have been included since they offer different types of knowing about reflection which are worthy of contemplation. In the last edition of this book I concentrated on reviewing the research on reflection in nursing (Bulman 2004). However, in this new edition it felt right to cast the net wider and consider some of the work from education research since I think it offers a perspective on reflection that nurses should take note of.

Nursing research

The nursing studies reviewed here range from 1989 to 2004 and focus on reflective education and practice. The majority of the studies were carried out in the UK. However, there were studies from Ireland, Hong Kong, Canada, Australia, New Zealand, the USA, the Netherlands and Finland, demonstrating the international interest in reflection amongst nurses, although there is a predominance of work within western society.

Outcomes of a reflective education

Significantly, studies appeared to indicate that reflective learning is a positive and useful experience for many students (McCaugherty 1991; Green and Holloway 1997; Hallet 1997; Smith 1998; Glaze 2001a,b; Paget 2001). There were also indications that reflection was a developmental process, with students reporting positive changes in their practice as they progressed through a reflective education programme (Durgahee 1996; Wong et al. 1997; Duke and Appleton 2000; Paget 2001). Furthermore, improved learning outcomes and greater success at assessment appeared to be demonstrated (Paget 2001). There was some evidence of the influence of reflection on qualified nurses' practice (Jasper 1999; Platzer et al. 2000a, 2000b; Glaze 2001a, 2001b; Paget 2001), but more work in this area would clearly be of interest.

Teachers' and students' experiences

There was a noticeable lack of attention given to how participants were prepared for reflective learning and how teachers were prepared for delivering a reflective curriculum (Hyrkas *et al.* 2001; Scanlan *et al.* 2002). There could also be a greater emphasis on researching the concerns and experiences of both students and teachers. Burnard (1995) and O'Connor *et al.* (2003), for instance, were the only ones reviewed who had attempted to capture the opinions and experiences of teachers. Burnard (1995) explored nurse teachers' perceptions of reflection. Although the majority of participants were positive and enthusiastic about reflection and teaching reflective practice, there were negative concerns surrounding its unproven value, exposing feelings and intimate values, time, difficulties of recollection and introspection. Participants were also vague about how reflection was actually taught to students and how it could improve clinical practice. This study was conducted some time ago and reflects a time when reflection was a new concept in nurse education. O'Connor *et al.*'s (2003) study is more recent and participants were certainly positive about the influences of reflection in the development of nursing knowledge. However, the research also suggested that teachers did not seem well prepared to facilitate reflection since some of the discourse revealed that they had little experience and limited knowledge of reflection.

There were some well-designed studies exploring students' experiences of reflection (Glaze 2001a,b; Paget 2001). Respondents in Paget's study felt that reflection did influence their clinical practice, helping them to learn how to learn. They described personal, broad and long-term changes and they continued to change after formal reflection and supervision had finished. Glaze's study also reported on MSc Advanced Nursing students' positive experiences of a reflective education. Students described developing greater awareness and appreciation of what nursing could be, becoming more realistic, open and confident, more assertive and enlightened, pushing the boundaries of practice, and this highlighted the desire to empower staff. Students found that reflection was a transformational process, which was demanding and influenced by their personal background.

Other studies highlighted many of the pros and cons inherent in teaching and learning about reflection. These included the benefits as well as the difficulties of group reflection and reflective writing as well as the lack of development in higher levels of critical thinking (Wong *et al.* 1997; Hayes 1998; Duke and Appleton 2000; Teekman 2000) and the use of reflection as a consciousness-raising tool (Durgahee 1996). The theme of powerlessness to change things despite a reflective education was also noteworthy (Duke and Appleton 2000; Graham 2000; Page and Meerabeau 2000; Paget 2001). These findings highlight the requirement to include planning and management of change as part of teaching about reflection and the need for a supportive and responsive clinical environment if reflective practice is to be encouraged. Mantzoukas and Jasper's (2004) fascinating ethnographic study particularly highlighted the contextual, social and political aspects surrounding the social construction of nursing and thus their effects on the successful and positive implementation of reflection into daily practice.

The influence of previous educational and life experiences was also raised by several studies (Mountford and Rogers 1996; Francis *et al.* 1998; Platzer *et al.* 2000a, 2000b; Glaze 2001a, 2001b) but was not explored in any depth. Many studies tended to focus on the development of cognitive aspects of reflection based on empirical factual knowledge, whilst some did overtly raise affective (emotional) and action (practical) issues (Powell 1989; Clarke and Graham 1996; Wallace 1996; Page and Meerabeau 2000). This is an area of research that needs more attention in relation to a concept of reflection as something more than rational thinking, as discussed earlier in the chapter.

Facilitating reflection

Many studies suggested that reflection takes time to develop, for example, Kember *et al.* (1996), Duke and Appleton (2000), Liimatainen *et al.* (2001) and Paget (2001). Consequently the requirement for good facilitation, challenge and support was emphasised by a number of studies, for example, Clarke and Graham (1996), Hayes (1998), Graham (2000), Platzer *et al.* (2000a,b) and Paget (2001). This has implications for curriculum development and the long-term commitment of mentoring and clinical support for reflection, and is further discussed in Chapters 4 and 5 of this book.

Assessing reflection

Importantly the difficulties of assessing reflection have not really been tackled by many studies and this remains an issue (Duke and Appleton 2000). The lack of well-validated tools for measuring levels of reflection was particularly evident from the research (Wong *et al.* 1997; Powell 1989; Duke and Appleton 2000) and makes the assumption, as Duke and Appleton commented, that there are levels of reflection which can be measured. Further exploration in this area is presented in Sue Schutz's chapter on assessing and evaluating reflection (Chapter 3).

A critique of the research

The nursing research reviewed was mainly qualitative, reflecting the need to explore an area in nursing where little previous work has been carried out. Nevertheless, there were some quantitative and combined method studies, for instance, Duke and Appleton (2000) and Paget (2001). Much of the research reviewed was small-scale and thus some may criticise the lack of generalisability in such work, although I would make the point here that the context and situatedness of some of this work on reflection is its strength, as I see it. Additionally, whilst the body of nursing research on reflection is growing, it still needs to be viewed tentatively, since a number of the papers lack information on their design.

It is worth noting that many studies were conducted by the same teachers who were also delivering the curriculum or were involved in some teaching capacity with the participants; this was also the case with the educational research reviewed. I would suggest that this has its roots in the teacher as researcher, promoted in educational research by Stenhouse from the 1970s, the lack of research funding for projects in this area, the enthusiasm of nurses to investigate the area, and thus the proliferation of many small-scale in-house studies. However, small studies should not automatically be dismissed but need to be conducted with rigor and with well-thought-out design if they are to add seriously to the body of research evidence (Heath 1998). Nevertheless there are power and value issues in relation to teachers researching their own students. Crucially, this includes the influence this has on what students are prepared to say and reveal to researchers who are also their teachers and presumably their assessors.

Despite initial criticisms of the nursing research to date, the work of Heath (1998) is again worthy of comment. She described the nursing literature as promoting the need for research that demonstrates large, quick benefits with measurable outcomes and that small accumulated gain is not considered valuable. Importantly, she suggested that the reality of knowledge development is often that evidence is built up by slow accumulation over time. So the promise of one large study in order to demonstrate that reflection makes a difference to client care is not a realistic option despite the repeated concern in the literature for the concept to demonstrate positive outcomes in client care (Heath 1998). However, Heath also suggested that the processes of care and outcome are complex and that the effect of reflection in terms of precise measurement and separation from other factors is difficult to achieve. Therefore she recommended the need to focus on the development of practitioners accepting the assumption that enhancing skills will lead to better patient care.

Nursing discussion papers

The literature contains a wealth of interesting discussion papers concerning reflection in nursing from the mid-1980s onwards; these papers are international with contributions from the UK, Australia and the USA. Those reviewed here were mainly written by nursing academics and those involved in teaching and supporting the development of reflection in nursing. Most strikingly, these papers represented divided camps about reflection amongst authors. There were some who were strongly critical of reflection, discussing the lack of an agreed definition, the lack of evidence that it makes any difference to patient care, and factors that affect effective reflection; for example, Newell (1994), Macintosh (1998), Burton (2000), Cotton (2001) and Burnard (2005). Whilst criticism about a lack of research evidence is justifiable, many of these papers appear to assume a stance that values only rational and propositional approaches to knowing.

There were also those papers that typified a more positive attitude towards reflection; for example, Clarke (1986), Jarvis (1992), Reid (1993), Johns (1995), Richardson (1995), Carr (1996) and Kim (1999). They discussed the benefits of learning from experience in order to develop personal as well as practical knowledge, characterised by Polanyi (1958), and focused on the need to take a critical look at practice. Hence these articles expressed a different view from those cited above. They demonstrated a shift in paradigm from rationality, objectivity and truth to a more interpretive approach to nursing; an approach seeking to understand and value personal and affective knowing and view it as as important as the rational and propositional (Johns 1995; Carr 1996).

Interestingly the papers that were more critical of reflection appeared later in the literature, seemingly confirming a backlash against earlier advocacy for reflection. In fact, Heath (1998) criticised the fact that debates in nursing do tend to be subject to inflexible paradigm positions intolerant of different standpoints, and this pattern can be seen in some of the discussion papers above. As Heath suggested, this indicates a requirement to debate strengths, limitations and uses rather than reject something outright or be totally uncritical and accepting of it. Her argument highlights the particular need for continued debate concerning the concept of reflection in nursing.

Clinical nursing papers

I have also included a snapshot of clinical nursing articles in this review (Laight 1995; Allan 1996; Edwards 1996; Ganner 1996; Gallichan 1997; Haddock and Bassett 1997; Ramsden 1997; Tarbrook 1997; Graham et al. 1998; McKenna 1999; Bekaert 2000; Kirrane 2001). These articles detail students' or qualified nurses' accounts of their practice. They explore nursing particular patients or general experiences of nursing practice and they all purport to use reflection to enhance this exploration. Whilst these articles would not be considered as evidence in the same way as research, they add to the exploration of the body of knowledge surrounding reflection. This is because they arose from nurses in practice trying to use reflection and they were published in journals that are read by practising nurses. Thus they are worthy of acknowledgement because of their link with practice. They show something of how reflection is being interpreted by nurses and not how it is being discussed by academics and theorists.

The articles demonstrate how the use of reflection gave the authors a means by which they could tell others about their practice experiences. There was evidence that nurses were using various reflective frameworks to achieve this, for example those by Boud *et al.* (1985) or Gibbs *et al.* (1988). This style of article seemed to be a replacement for the traditional 'case study' clinical article where the author presented and objectively discussed a 'nursing case', the discussion of thoughts and feelings about practice not traditionally part of this type of case study approach.

The reflective articles reviewed still focus on patients and practice but offer an additional element, because nurses were writing their thoughts and feelings about the complexities of their practice rather than following a purely objective/propositional approach. These papers are often characterised by description of thoughts and feelings about practice without critical reflection. In fact, there is a noticeable lack of reflection demonstrating critical analysis, echoing the research findings above. The articles reveal practice experiences and personal generation of knowledge about practice, which would not necessarily appear in a more traditional nursing text. They appear to be a vehicle for 'storytelling' about practice, but it is evident that they are not always critical. There is no suggestion of authors receiving coaching or facilitation for their reflection in most of the examples, with only one article (an MSc study) making explicit reference to facilitation of reflection in a group (Kirrane 2001).

This part of the review demonstrates a change in how knowing about practice was being communicated in published form, in a way that has begun to appreciate the affective and active knowledge about practice as well as the cognitive. It is evident that the nature of this knowledge could not always be described as critical, although it did seem to offer a route for nurses to 'tell their stories' about practice in ways that have not always been previously seen in the nursing literature.

A concise look at education literature and some comparisons with nursing

A review of the education literature reveals a great deal of interest and work around reflection during the 1980s and continuing today. The work is dominated by studies and educational projects from the USA and seems to have been influenced by a movement towards a more autonomous, questioning teacher as a reaction to the social and political pressure to control and regulate education in the United States (Zeichner and Liston 1987; Zeichner 1993). This was completely different to the research in nursing where work was dominated by British and Australasian papers, with very little work emerging from the USA. In similar ways to the nursing research reviewed, many of the education papers do not give detail about the design of their studies. Instead educationalists appeared to relish the cut and trust of the educational debate that arose from their work, rather than necessarily focusing on describing the details of their design. Good examples include the work of Wubbels and Korthagen (1990), Tann (1993), Newell (1996) and Dinkelmann (2000). There is also a predominance of work that described and analysed reflective education programmes but that was not necessarily presented as research. In a similar way to the clinical nursing papers, these are valuable to review because they were generated by teachers writing about their practice.

Literature in the area particularly focused on finding solutions to developing reflection in students (Ashcroft and Griffiths 1989; Maher in Tabachnich and Zeichner 1991; Guillaume and Rudney 1993; Valli 1993; Clarke 1995; Jay and Johnson 2002). Korthagen and Wubbels (1995) also identified issues and problems to be overcome and attempted to isolate attributes and correlates of the reflective practitioner; these are further illustrated in the next chapter of this book on skills and attributes for reflection. Again, this has similarities with nursing research where researchers are focusing on the development of a reflective curriculum and its outcomes.

Facilitation of reflection

Evidence suggested the need for expert facilitation of reflection in both pre-service students (Zeichner and Liston 1987; Ashcroft and Griffiths 1989; Reilly Freese 1999) and post-experience teachers (Newell 1996). Ashcroft (1992) particularly raised the issues of Plato's paradox of learning in relation to this, emphasising the need for expert facilitation in reflection due to the difficulties of knowing what one does not know and recognising this when one has found it. Plato's Paradox of Learning proposed that certain things are unlearnable because they must be known before any process of learning could take place (Honderich 1995). The research also pinpointed a practical issue around the use and expertise of practice supervisors and mentor-teachers. Similarly to mentors in nursing, these individuals appeared to have a lack of status and recognition, operated in different ways and also required support and co-ordination (Zeichner and Liston 1987; Manoucherii 2002).

Levels of reflection

Work on the levels of reflection has also been generated from well-known education research (Mezirow 1981; Goodman 1984; Carr and Kemmis 1986). However, Zeichner (1993) advised against thinking about the development of students in terms of so-called *levels of reflection*. Instead he called for the requirement to look at these as *domains of reflection* where each is important and necessary. Interestingly, some nursing research (Powell 1989; Wong et al. 1997) has taken up the use of these levels of reflection but without the same level of criticism demonstrated by Zeichner above. Work by Mezirow and Goodman on levels of reflection is further presented in Chapter 9.

Reflection over time

Education papers also raised the need to explore reflection, not simply focusing on an incident but an exploration of how reflection extends and interweaves across time and situations (Clarke 1995). This appears to fit with Jarvis et al.'s (2003) suggestions about the nature of experience. They defined experience as an ambiguous concept, being both lifelong and episodic. So, for example, we can have direct experiences but they can be qualified and modified by previous experiences. This points to the notion of our experiences being constructed, and thus as Jarvis et al. say, every experience is in some sense 'real' even if it is indirect or mediated.

This may indicate why research on reflective education programmes thus far reveals mixed success in demonstrating the development of reflection in education students and a lack of apparent belief in changes about their teaching. Indeed, educationalists such as Maher (1991) and Calderhead and Gates (1993) indicated that the legacy of reflection *may only be seen in the long term* or *when one's beliefs are seriously challenged* (Maher 1991; Calderhead and Gates 1993). However, as in nursing research, there is some evidence that students do value reflection or at least come to see its value in time (Zeichner and Liston 1987; Guillame and Rudney 1993; Newell 1996).

Concepts of reflection

In particular the education literature shows that concepts of reflection vary between educationalists (Grimmett and Erickson 1988; Calderhead and Gates 1993; Zeichner 1993). Significantly, educational literature emphasises the need to marry organisational goals with goals for reflection (Zeichner and Liston 1987; Valli in Calderhead and Gates 1993; Korthagen and Wubbels 1995). This suggests that educationalists' definitions of reflection will differ depending on the social factors influencing the educational organisation and collaborating practice areas. This certainly has significance for nursing, where each organisation would presumably need to look at what its expectations of reflection are and to share and develop this with other organisations. Barnett (1992) also commented on the lack of agreed meaning concerning reflection amongst educationalists in higher education. He suggested that there was not the same debate regarding critical thinking, which is privileged and also interpreted by people in slightly different ways. This is an important point; critical thinking has a long legacy of acceptance and consequently is not subjected to the same scrutiny as the relatively new concept of reflection.

Despite this lack of agreement it is still possible to see the influence of rationality in educationalists' interpretations of reflection, even when they purport to appreciate the intermingling of action, emotion and rationality in the process of reflection (Zeichner and Liston 1987; Ashcroft in Biott and Niass 1992; Valli in Calderhead and Gates 1993; Zeichner 1993; Clarke 1995; Korthagen and Wubbels 1995; Parker 1997; Usher *et al.* 1997; Brockbank and McGill 1998). Again, this has similarities with some of the nursing discussion papers mentioned above. Additionally, Parker (1997) and Usher *et al.* (1997) went as far as to critique reflective practice as a variation on the theme of realism and to criticise the continuing dominance of a rationalist framework, where reason rather than sense experience is the foundation of certainty in knowledge, despite reflection purporting to offer something different. Interestingly, very little education work extrapolated the influences of emotion on reflection, although Noddings (1984) has generated some interest in educationalists in her urge to value the affective as complementary to rationality and necessary for moral and ethical thinking.

It was also possible to see the influence of the critical theorists on educationalists' views of reflection (Van Manen 1977; Carr and Kemmis 1986; Zeichner and Liston 1987). However, there was little evidence that students were able to critically reflect on their practice, taking into account the broader issues of social, cultural, political and historical interest. In fact, they appeared to focus more on themselves and the immediate concerns they had for surviving in the classroom (Zeichner and Liston 1987; Dinkelmann 2000; Jay and Johnson 2002). This may well be the case with inexperienced nursing students and is suggested by Burrows (1995) within the nursing literature.

A change of research focus

Finally I think it is of interest that education research on reflection particularly indicates the need to pay attention to language (Russell *et al.* 1988; Weil and McGill 1989; Calderhead and Gates 1993; Tann 1993; Valli 1993). This debate highlights the need to focus on what practitioners are reflecting on, how they are going about it and what influences their reflection (Zeichner 1993; Parker 1997; Usher *et al.* 1997). There appears to be a shift of emphasis in the literature from focusing on development of the reflective curriculum to how people make sense of their experience through constructions of meaning (Denzin and Lincoln 2000). This is something that I believe research in nursing needs to pay some attention to. Thus greater focus on the process of reflection and on its social construction seems to me to be significant in understanding its further development in nursing.

Conclusion

I hope this introductory chapter has begun to give you an idea of what reflection is, as well as encouraging you to regard it with a critical eye. I believe that with constructive support and challenge, reflection can help nurses to get to grips with making sense of their experiences, as well as providing a route to encourage them to value their practical knowing and continue to develop it in a positive way. Getting prepared by reading about reflection, as you have just done, is a good start in obtaining an initial grasp of the concept. However, now you need to have a go at doing it – whether this involves designing a curriculum that supports reflection or doing some research or taking it forward with your work colleagues, depending on your reasons for reading this book. In essence, give it a go and find out what it can offer you.

References

Allan, H. (1996) Developing nursing knowledge and language. *Nursing Standard*, **10** (50), 42–44.

Ashcroft, K. (1992) Working together: developing reflective student teachers. In: *Working and Learning Together for Change. Developing Teachers and Teaching* (eds C. Biott and J. Niass). Open University Press, Buckingham.

Ashcroft, K. and Griffiths, M. (1989) Reflective teachers and reflective tutors: school experience in an initial teacher education course. *Journal of Education for Teaching*, **15** (1), 35–52.

Atkins, S. and Murphy, C. (1993) Reflection: a review of the literature. *Journal of Advanced Nursing*, **18** (8), 1188–1192.

Barnett, R. (1992) *Improving Higher Education*. Society for Research into Higher Education/Open University Press, London.

Barnett, R. (1997) *Higher Education: A Critical Business*. Society for Research into Higher Education/Open University Press, London.

Bekaert, S. (2000) Reflection on practice: a student perspective. *Paediatric Nursing*, **12** (1), 6–7.

Bloor, D. (1983) *Wittgenstein. A Social Theory of Knowledge*. Macmillan Education, London.

Boud, D., Keogh, R. and Walker, D. (1985) *Reflection: Turning Learning into Experience*. Kogan Page, London.

Boyd, E.M. and Fales, A.W. (1983) Reflective learning: key to learning from experience. *Journal of Humanistic Psychology*, **23** (2), 99–117.

Brookfield, S.D. (1987) *Developing Critical Thinkers. Challenging Adults to Explore Alternative Ways of Thinking*. Jossey Bass, San Francisco.

Bulman, C. (2004) An introduction to reflection. In: *Reflective Practice in Nursing. The Growth of the Professional Practitioner* (eds C. Bulman and S. Schutz), 3rd edn. Blackwell Scientific Publications, Oxford.

Burnard, P. (1995) Nurse educators' perceptions of reflection and reflective practice: a report of a descriptive study. *Journal of Advanced Nursing*, **21**, 1167–1174.

Burnard, P. (2005) Reflections on reflection (Editorial). *Nurse Education Today*, **25**, 85–86.

Burrows, D. (1995) The nurse teacher's role in the promotion of reflective practice. *Nurse Education Today*, **15**, 346–350.

Burton, A.J. (2000) Reflection: nursing's practice and education panacea? *Journal of Advanced Nursing*, **31** (5), 1009–1017.

Brockbank, A. and McGill, I. (1998) *Facilitating Reflective Learning in Higher Education*. Society for Research into Higher Education/Open University Press, London.

Calderhead, J. and Gates, P. (1993) (eds) *Conceptualising Reflection in Teacher Development*. The Falmer Press, London.

Canfield, J.V. (1986) *The Philosophy of Wittgenstein. Volume 12. Persons*. Garland Publishing, New York.

Carr, E. (1996) Reflecting on clinical practice: hectoring talk or reality? *Journal of Clinical Nursing*, **5**, 289–295.

Carr, W. and Kemmis, S. (1986) *Becoming Critical: Education, Knowledge and Action Research*. The Falmer Press, London.

Champion, R. (1992) The philosophy of an honours degree programme in nursing and midwifery. In: *Developing Professional Education* (eds H. Bines and D. Watson). Society for Research into Higher Education/Open University Press, London.

Clarke, A. (1995) Professional development in practicum settings: reflective practice under scrutiny. *Teaching and Teacher Education*, **11** (3), 243–261.

Clarke, B., James, C. and Kelly, J. (1996) Reflective practice: reviewing the issues and refocusing the debate. *International Journal of Nursing Studies*, **33** (20), 181–189.

Clarke, D.J. and Graham, M. (1996) Reflective practice, the use of reflective diaries by experienced registered nurses. *Nursing Review*, **15** (1), 26–29.

Clarke, M. (1986) Action and reflection: practice and theory in nursing. *Journal of Advanced Nursing*, **11**, 3–11.

Clift, R.T., Houston, W.R. and Pugach, M.C. (1990) (eds) *Encouraging Reflective Practice in Education. An Analysis of Issues and Programs*. Teachers' College Press, Columbia University, New York.

Clinton, M. (1998) On reflection in action: unaddressed issues in re-focusing the debate in reflective practice. *International Journal of Nursing Practice*, **4** (30), 197–203.

Cottingham, J. (1997) *Descartes' Philosophy of the Mind*. Phoenix, London.

Cotton, A.H. (2001) Private thoughts in public spheres: issues in reflection and reflective practices in nursing. *Journal of Advanced Nursing*, **36** (4), 512–519.

Day, J.M. (1994) (ed.) *Plato's Meno in Focus*. Routledge, London.

Denzin, N.K. and Lincoln, Y.S. (eds) (2000) *Handbook of Qualitative Research*. Sage, London.

Dewey, J. (1933) *How We Think. A Restatement of the Relation of Reflective Thinking to the Educative Process*. DC Heath, Boston.

Dinkelmann, T. (2000) An inquiry into the development of critical reflection in secondary student teachers. *Teaching and Teacher Education*, **16**, 195–229.

Duke, S. (2000) The experience of becoming reflective In: *Reflective Practice in Nursing. The Growth of the Professional Practitioner* (eds S. Burns and C. Bulman), 2nd edn. Blackwell Scientific Publications, Oxford.

Duke, S. and Appleton, J. (2000) The use of reflection in a palliative care programme: a quantitative study of reflective skills over an academic year. *Journal of Advanced Nursing*, **32** (6), 1557–1568.

Durgahee, T. (1996) Promoting reflection in postgraduate nursing: a theoretical model. *Nurse Education Today*, **16**, 419–426.

Edwards, M. (1996) Patient–nurse relationships: using reflective practice. *Nursing Standard*, **10** (25), 40–43.

Eraut, M. (1994) *Developing Professional Knowledge and Competence*. The Falmer Press, London.

FitzGerald, M. and Chapman, Y. (2000) Theories of reflection for learning. In: *Reflective Practice in Nursing. The Growth of the Professional Practitioner* (eds S. Burns and C. Bulman), 2nd edn. Blackwell Scientific Publications, Oxford.

Francis, D., Owens, J. and Tollefson, J. (1998) 'It comes together at the end': the impact of a one-year subject in nursing inquiry on philosophies of nursing. *Nursing Inquiry*, **5**, 268–278.

Freire, P. (1972) *Pedagogy of the Oppressed*. Herder and Herder, New York.

Gallichan, M. (1997) Reflective practice. *Nursing Times*, **93** (26), 57.

Ganner, C. (1996) Using reflection in a critical care unit. *Nursing Standard*, **10** (15), 23–26.

Gibbs, G., Farmer, B. and Eastcott, D. (1988) *Learning by Doing. A Guide to Teaching and Learning Methods*, pp. 46–47. FEU, Birmingham Polytechnic.

Glaze, J. (2001a) Reflection as a transforming process: student advanced nurse practitioners' experiences on developing reflective skills as part of an MSc programme. *Journal of Advanced Nursing*, **34** (5), 639–647.

Glaze, J. (2001b) Stages in coming to terms with reflection: student advanced nurse practitioners' perceptions of their reflective journeys. *Journal of Advanced Nursing*, **37** (3), 265–272.

Goodman, J. (1984) Reflection and teacher education: a case study and theoretical analysis. *Interchange*, **15** (3), 9–26.

Graham, I., Waight, S. and Scammel, J. (1998) Using structured reflection to improve nursing practice. *Nursing Times*, **94** (25), 56–59.

Graham, I.W. (2000) Reflective practice and its role in mental health nurses' practice development: a year long study. *Journal of Psychiatric and Mental Health Nursing*, **7**, 109–117.

Green, A.J. and Holloway, D.G. (1997) Using a phenomenological research technique to examine student nurses' understandings of experiential teaching and learning: a critical review of methodological issues. *Journal of Advanced Nursing*, **26**, 1013–1019.

Grimmett, P.P. and Erickson, G.L. (eds) (1988) *Reflection in Teacher Education*. Teachers' College Press, New York, and Pacific Educational Press, Vancouver.

Guillaume, A.M. and Rudney, G.L. (1993) Student teachers' growth towards independence: an analysis of their changing concerns. *Teaching and Teacher Education*, **9** (1), 65–80.

Hacker, P.M.S. (1997) *Wittgenstein*. Phoenix, London.

Haddock, J. and Bassett, C. (1997) Nurses' perceptions of reflective practice. *Nursing Standard*, **11** (32), 39–41.

Hallett, C.E. (1997) Learning through reflection in the community: the relevance of Schön's theories of coaching to nursing education. *International Journal of Nursing Studies*, **34** (2), 103–110.

Hayes, J. (1998) Learning from practice: developing the reflective skills of forensic psychiatric nurses. *Psychiatric Care*, **5** (1), 30–33.

Heath, H. (1998) Paradigm dialogues and dogma: finding a place for research, nursing models and reflective practice. *Journal of Advanced Nursing*, **28** (2), 288–294.

Honderich, T. (1995) *The Oxford Companion to Philosophy*. Oxford University Press, Oxford.

Hyrkas, K., Tarkka, M.T. and Paunonen-Ilmonen, M. (2001) Teacher candidates' reflective teaching and learning in a hospital setting – changing the pattern of practical training: a challenge to growing into teacher-hood. *Journal of Advanced Nursing*, **33** (4), 503–511.

James, C.R. and Clarke, B.A. (1994) Reflective practice in nursing: issues and implications for nursing education. *Nurse Education Today*, **14**, 82–90.

Jarvis, P. (1983) *Professional Education*. Croom Helm, London.

Jarvis, P. (1992) Reflective practice and nursing. *Nurse Education Today*, **12**, 174–181.

Jarvis, P., Holford, J. and Griffin, C. (eds) (2003) *The Theory and Practice of Learning*. Kogan Page, London.

Jasper, M.A. (1999) Nurses' perceptions of the value of written reflection. *Nurse Education Today*, **19**, 452–463.

Jay, J.K. and Johnson, K.L. (2002) Capturing complexity: a typology of reflective practice for teacher education. *Teaching and Teacher Education*, **18,** 73–85.

Johns, C. (1995) The value of reflective practice for nursing. *Journal of Clinical Nursing*, **4**, 23–30.

Johns, C. (2000) *Becoming a Reflective Practitioner. A Reflective and Holistic Approach to Clinical Nursing, Practice Development and Clinical Supervision*. Blackwell Science, Oxford.

Kember, D., Jones, A., Loke, A., *et al.* (1996) Developing curricula to encourage students to write reflective journals. *Educational Action Research*, **4** (3), 329–348.

Kim, H.S. (1999) Critical reflective inquiry for knowledge development in nursing practice. *Journal of Advanced Nursing*, **29** (5), 1205–1212.

Kirrane, C. (2001) Using action learning in reflective practice. *Professional Nurse*, **16** (5), 1102–1105.

Korthagen, F.A.J. and Wubbels, T. (1995) Characteristics of reflective practitioners: towards an operationalisation of the concept of reflection. *Teachers and Teaching: Theory and Practice*, **1** (1), 51–72.

Laight, S. (1995) The aggressive ward visitor: a critical incident analysis. *Nursing Times*, **91** (48), 40–41.

Liimatainen, L., Poskiparta, M., Karhila, P. and Sjogren, A. (2001) The development of reflective learning in the context of health counseling and health promotion during nurse education. *Journal of Advanced Nursing*, **34** (5), 648–658.

Mackintosh, C. (1998) Reflection: a flawed strategy for the nursing profession. *Nurse Education Today*, **18**, 553–557.

Maher, F. (1991) Reflexivity and teacher education: the Wheaton programme. In: *Issues and Practices in Inquiry Orientated Teacher Education* (eds B.R. Tabachnich and K. Zeichner). The Falmer Press, London.

Manoucherii, A. (2002) Developing teaching knowledge through peer discourse. *Teaching and Teacher Education*, **18**, 715–737.

Mantzoukas, S. and Jasper, M.A. (2004) Reflective practice and daily ward reality: a covert power game. *Journal of Clinical Nursing*, **13**, 913–924.

McCaugherty, D. (1991) The use of a teaching model to promote reflection and the experiential integration of theory and practice in first-year student nurses: an action research project. *Journal of Advanced Nursing*, **16**, 534–543.

McKenna, H. (1999) The role of reflection in the development of practice theory: a case study. *Journal of Psychiatric and Mental Health Nursing*, **6** (2), 147–151.

McMahon, R. and Pearson, A. (eds) (1998) *Nursing as Therapy*, 2nd edn. Stanley Thornes, Cheltenham.

Mezirow, J. (1981) A critical theory of adult learning and education. *Adult Education*, **32** (1), 3–24.

Mountford, B. and Rogers, L. (1996) Using individual and group reflection in and on assessment as a tool for effective learning. *Journal of Advanced Nursing*, **24**, 1127–1134.

Mulhall, A. and Le May, A. (1999) Bridging the research–practice gap: a reflective account of research work. *Nursing Times Research*, **4** (2), 119–129.

Newell, R. (1994) Reflection: art, science or pseudo-science. Guest Editorial. *Nurse Education Today*, **14**, 79–81.

Newell, S.T. (1996) Practical inquiry: collaboration and reflection in teacher education reform. *Teaching and Teacher Education*, **12** (6), 567–576.

Noddings, N. (1984) *Caring. A Feminine Approach to Ethics and Moral Education*. University of California Press, Berkeley.

Nursing and Midwifery Council (2004a) *Standards of Proficiency for Pre-registration Nurse Education*. NMC, London.

Nursing and Midwifery Council (2004b) *Standards for the Preparation of Teachers of Nurses, Midwives and Specific Community Public Health Nurses*. NMC, London.

Nursing and Midwifery Council (2004c) *Supporting Nurses and Midwives Through Lifelong Learning*. NMC, London.

Nursing and Midwifery Council (2005) *The PREP Handbook*. NMC, London.

O'Connor, A., Hyde, A. and Treacey, M. (2003) Nurse teachers' constructions of reflection and reflective practice. Qualitative research into tutors' perceptions and experiences of using reflection with diploma nursing students in Ireland. *Reflective Practice*, **2**, 107–119.

Page, S. and Meerabeau, L. (2000) Achieving change through reflective practice: closing the loop. *Nurse Education Today*, **20**, 365–372.

Paget, T. (2001) Reflective practice and clinical outcomes: practitioners' views on how reflective practice has influenced their clinical practice. *Journal of Clinical Nursing*, **10**, 204–214.

Parker, S. (1997) *Reflective Teaching in the Post-Modern World – A Manifesto for Education in Post-modernity*. Open University Press, Buckingham.

Paterson, J.G. and Zderad, L.T. (1988) *Humanistic Nursing*. National League for Nursing, New York.

Platzer, H., Blake, D. and Ashford, D. (2000a) Barriers to learning from reflection: a study of the use of group work with post registration students. *Journal of Advanced* Nursing, **31** (5), 1001–1008.

Platzer, H., Blake, D. and Ashford, D. (2000b) An evaluation of process and outcomes from learning through reflective practice groups on a post-registration nursing course. *Journal of Advanced Nursing*, **31** (3), 689–695.

Polanyi, M. (1958) *Personal Knowledge*. Routledge and Keegan Paul, London.

Polanyi, M. (1967) *The Tacit Dimension*. Doubleday, New York.

Powell, J. (1989) The reflective practitioner in nursing. *Journal of Advanced Nursing*, **14**, 824–832.

Ramsden, J. (1997) Objective analysis of a critical incident. *Nursing Times*, **93** (34), 43–45.

Reed, J. and Ground, I. (1997) *Philosophy for Nursing*. Arnold, London.

Reid, B. (1993) 'But we're doing it already!' Exploring a response to the concept of reflective practice in order to improve its facilitation. *Nurse Education Today*, **13**, 305–309.

Reilley Freese, A. (1999) The role of reflection on preservice teachers' development in the context of a professional development school. *Teaching and Teacher Education*, **15**, 895–909.

Richardson, R. (1995) Humpty Dumpty: reflection and reflective nursing practice. *Journal of Advanced Nursing*, **21**, 1044–1050.

Rogers, C. (1983) *Freedom to Learn for the 80s*. Charles Merrill, Columbus, Ohio.

Russell, T., Munby, H., Spafford, C. and Johnston, P. (1988) Learning the professional knowledge of teaching: metaphors, puzzles and the theory–practice relationship. In: *Reflection in Teacher Education* (eds D.P. Grimmett and G.L. Erickson). Teachers' College Press, New York, and Pacific Educational Press, Vancouver.

Ryle, G. (1963) *The Concept of the Mind*. Penguin, Harmondsworth.

Ryle, G. (1979) *On Thinking*. Blackwell, Oxford.

Saylor, C. (1990) Reflection and professional education: art, science and competency. *Nurse Educator*, **15** (2), 8–11.

Scanlan, J.M., Dean Care, W. and Udod, S. (2002) Unraveling the unknowns of reflection in classroom teaching. *Journal of Advanced Nursing*, **38** (2), 136–143.

Schön, D.A. (1983) *The Reflective Practitioner*. Basic Books, Harper Collins, San Francisco.

Schön, D.A. (1987) *Educating the Reflective Practitioner*. Jossey Bass, San Francisco.

Schön, D.A. (1992) *The Reflective Practitioner*, 2nd edn. Jossey Bass, San Francisco.

Smith, A. (1998) Learning about reflection. *Journal of Advanced Nursing*, **28** (4), 891–898.

Tann, S. (1993) Eliciting student teachers' personal theories. In: *Conceptualising Reflection in Teacher Development* (eds J. Calderhead and P. Gates). The Falmer Press, London.

Tarbrook, D. (1997) Students. On the rebound. *Nursing Times*, **93** (50), 60–62.

Teekman, B. (2000) Exploring reflective thinking in nursing practice. *Journal of Advanced Nursing*, **31** (5), 1125–1135.

United Kingdom Central Council for Nursing and Midwifery (1994) *The Future of Professional Practice. The Council's Standards for Education and Practice Following Registration.* UKCC, London.

United Kingdom Central Council for Nursing and Midwifery (1996) PREP and you – your guide to profiling. *Register*, **17**, 7–10.

Usher, R., Bryant, I. and Johnston, R. (1997) *Adult Education and the Post-Modern Challenge. Learning Beyond the Limits.* Routledge, London.

Valli, L.R. (1993) Reflective teacher education programmes: an analysis of case studies. In: *Conceptualising Reflection in Teacher Development* (J.G. Calderhead and P. Gates). The Falmer Press, London.

Van Manen, M. (1977) Linking ways of knowing with ways of being practical. *Curriculum Inquiry*, **6** (3), 205–228.

Wallace, D. (1996) Experiential learning and critical thinking in nursing. *Nursing Standard*, **10** (31), 43–47.

Weil, S.W. and McGill, I. (eds) (1989) *Making Sense of Experiential Learning: Diversity in Theory and Practice.* Society for Research into Higher Education/ Open University Press, London.

Wittgenstein, L. (1967) *Philosophical Investigations.* Blackwell, Oxford.

Wong, F.K.Y., Loke, A.Y.L., Wong, M., Tse, H., Kan, E. and Kember, D. (1997) An action research study into the development of nurses as reflective practitioners. *Journal of Nursing Education*, **36** (10), 476 – 481.

Wubbels, T. and Korthagen, F.A.J. (1990) The effects of a pre-service teacher education program for the preparation of reflective teachers. *Journal of Education for Teaching*, **16** (1), 29–43.

Zeichner, K.M. (1993) Connecting genuine teacher development to the struggle for social justice. *Journal of Education for Teaching*, **19** (1), 5–20.

Zeichner, K.M. and Liston, D.P. (1987) Teaching student teachers to reflect. *Harvard Educational Review*, **57** (1), 23–48.

Chapter 2

Developing the skills for reflective practice

Sue Atkins and Sue Schutz

Introduction

This chapter is based upon an assumption that there are certain skills underlying the development and use of reflective practice. During the past 15 years, there has been much discussion and debate within nursing and health care literature about the nature of reflection and how reflective practice may be facilitated in professional courses (Clarke *et al.* 1996; Greenwood 1998; Boud 1999; Burton 2000; Hannigan 2001). A number of small research studies have been undertaken to investigate reflective learning in nursing, for example Durgahee (1998), Jasper (1999) and Page and Meerabeau (2000). It is now widely understood that reflective practice is a process of learning and development through examining one's own practice including experiences, thoughts, feelings, actions and knowledge (Mezirow 1981; Brockbank and McGill 1998; Kim 1999; Bolton 2005). These and other authors emphasise that reflection involves reviewing one's own values, challenging assumptions and considering broader social, political and professional issues that are relevant but may be beyond personal practice experience. The latter is essential if reflection is to result in significant and positive social change.

An earlier review of key literature on reflection from the fields of education and critical social theory suggested that the skills of *self-awareness, description, critical analysis, synthesis* and *evaluation* are necessary to engage in reflective practice (Atkins and Murphy 1993). The purpose of this chapter is to explore these skills and present a series of exercises aimed at helping nurses and other health and social care professionals to examine, develop and refine their skills. We also offer an alternative perspective of developing reflective practice which may be useful for more experienced practitioners. It is evident that the deliberate and systematic use of reflection as a learning tool in professional practice is a complex activity that needs to be consciously developed by pre- and post-qualifying professionals over time (Burrows 1995; Glaze 2001; Duke and Appleton 2000; Bulman and Schutz 2004; Johns and Freshwater

2005). It is also widely acknowledged that the development of reflective learning and practice requires skilled, sensitive facilitation, and appropriate guidance and support from educators, supervisors and mentors (Brockbank and McGill 1998; Johns 2000; Paget 2001). A variety of approaches are used to facilitate reflection. These include the use of models and structured frameworks (for example, Gibbs *et al.* 1988; Johns 2005), reflective writing and the use of journals (Paterson 1995; Bolton 2005), engaging in reflective dialogue (Brockbank and McGill 1998; Bolton 2005), and the use of action learning sets (McGill and Beaty 2001). The intention of the skills-based approach, presented in this chapter, is to complement these approaches and to work with them.

A series of exercises is presented, for use by practitioners and facilitators, with a separate section devoted to each skill. The meaning of the skill is defined and explored, highlighting its relevance for both professional practice and academic work. The importance of each skill for reflective practice is justified with reference to key theories and recent research. The exercises enable participants to practise the skills of reflection alone, with a colleague or friend or within a group. In practice and in education, the importance of combining individual and group activity in the development of reflective learning is supported by research studies, for example Durgahee (1996) and Wong *et al.* (1997). In particular, the value of engaging in reflective dialogue with others in order to achieve deeper levels of reflection is apparent. In this edition, we also present a section that outlines and discusses the attributes of reflective practice, with a view to development of these in experienced practitioners.

The importance of underlying skills

An examination of the nature and process of reflective practice, as discussed by key and influential theorists, for example Mezirow (1981), Schön (1983) and Boud *et al.* (1985), suggests that there are underlying skills involved in reflective practice. The skills of self-awareness, description, critical analysis, synthesis and evaluation are implicit in the models and theories of these authors. For example, in Boud *et al.*'s (1985) analysis of the reflective process, the need to attend to feelings and attitudes, in particular making use of positive feelings and dealing with negative feelings, is apparent throughout, and requires self-awareness. The stages labelled as *Association, Integration, Validation* and *Appropriation* involve varying degrees of critical analysis, synthesis and evaluation. Similarly, if one takes Mezirow's (1981) concept of reflectivity and studies its seven different dimensions or levels, it is clear that self-awareness is integral at all levels. The need for description, analysis, synthesis and evaluation becomes more evident when moving up the hierarchy from *Discriminant* to *Theoretical Reflectivity*. Schön's (1983) analysis of the reflective practitioner's use of 'reflection-on-action' and 'reflection-in-action' implies the use of similar skills.

More recently, the development of structured models and frameworks to guide reflective practice in nursing education makes the use of these skills more explicit (2005 Duke and Appleton 2000; Johns 2005). The importance of these underlying skills has been reinforced by a number of small-scale research projects that examine the development of reflection in students undertaking pre- and post-qualifying nursing courses (Wong *et al.* 1997; Jasper 1999; Duke and Appleton 2000; Glaze 2001; Paget 2001). Jasper's grounded theory study identified reflective writing as an important strategy for developing self-awareness and critical analysis. Duke and Appleton's quantitative study of palliative care students' development of reflective skills over an academic year demonstrated that reflective skills are developed over time, and that the higher-level skills necessary for critical reflection are harder to develop and take longer to achieve. In Glaze's exploratory study of student advanced nurse practitioners' experiences of developing reflective skills, the practitioners describe their deepening self-awareness, greater critical analysis abilities (especially in relation to socio-political issues), and their efforts at synthesis and evaluation through attempts to empower colleagues and bring about changes in practice.

It is interesting to note that there are similarities between the skills underlying reflective practice and the skills required for academic study. With the exception of self-awareness, these underlying skills are the higher order cognitive or thinking skills identified within Bloom *et al.*'s (1956) taxonomy of educational objectives. This taxonomy or hierarchy has guided and influenced the development of leaning programmes, objectives and outcomes within higher education. Therefore, developing and refining these underlying skills may not only help to develop a more reflective style of practice, but also further the development of academic skills and ability to integrate theory with practice. This is especially important for people undertaking work-based learning and professional development courses and also for practice development.

Limitations of a skills-based approach to developing reflective practice

It is important to acknowledge the limitations of a skills-based approach to developing reflectivity. As we have seen earlier, reflective skills are acquired and developed gradually through practice over time, rather than in any one course or package. While these exercises involve reflecting on practice, frequently away from the clinical setting, it is important to acknowledge that reflective practice, most importantly, is a way of examining thoughts, feelings and actions while actually *engaged in professional practice*, as illustrated in Schön's (1983) work. Greenwood (1998) also introduced the notion of reflection before action, an idea that has yet to be developed and remains controversial. People have individual styles of learning and may learn in different ways, depending upon their personality, maturity and experience. Therefore, the extent to which individuals may find the skills-based approach to developing reflective practice presented in this chapter to be helpful is likely to vary. Highly structured and staged approaches to developing skills for reflective practice may be more suitable for less experienced students on pre-registration programmes, as indicated by the work of Burrows (1995). It has been suggested by Bolton (2005) that the use of structured frameworks and exercises may be restrictive and counter-productive to the development of creativity in professional practice. Bolton (2005) advocates a less structured, narrative approach whereby practitioners write freely about their practice experiences and share their writing within a facilitated group.

It is apparent that other skills, not addressed in this chapter, are also important, especially when engaging in reflection with other people. These include skills of active listening, empathy, assertiveness, supporting and challenging and the planning and management of change (Brockbank and McGill 1998; Durgahee 1998; Page and Meerabeau 2000). In particular, change management skills are important if the outcome of reflection is to have a positive impact on practice. It is recommended that readers consult some of the many texts available on change management.

A wide-ranging approach to developing reflective practice

For more experienced practitioners, and for those of you who find a skills-based approach does not suit you, you could consider some of the work that has been done to define a wider approach to reflective practice. In our work, we have carefully considered the writing of Schön (1983, 1987) and have discerned some characteristics or attributes of reflective practice from his work. These open up the notion of the reflective practitioner rather more than the skills-based approach does and views the concept of reflective practice as something that can develop over time, possibly without specific action from the practitioner and is, perhaps, more personal. Having said this, thoughtful and purposeful practice in nursing includes active consideration of development towards reflective practice and such attributes do not 'come to us' automatically. Through participation in academic and practice-based courses, through reflection, supervision and through self-awareness, the experienced practitioner can develop these attributes.

If you are already engaged in reflection and would like to enhance your skills further, we suggest that you turn to the section entitled 'Attributes of the reflective practitioner' at the end of this chapter.

Guidance on using the exercises in this chapter

In this chapter, three types of exercises are presented. They are:

- *On-your-own exercises*: these are exercises that you can undertake alone, without a facilitator. It is recommended that about 15–30 minutes be spent on each of these exercises.
- *With-a-partner exercises*: these you should try with a colleague or fellow student. These exercises will take approximately 30–60 minutes.
- *With-a-group exercises*: these are designed to be undertaken in a group with a facilitator. These exercises will take about 30–90 minutes.

All exercises require a commitment of time and thought, just as reflection does. Taking the exercises slowly over several weeks is recommended as the best approach. It will also be helpful to refer to the many examples and extracts of reflection within other chapters of this book.

Issues for facilitators

It is recommended that facilitators be educators or supervisors who are experienced and feel comfortable working with adult learners. Facilitators are reminded of the importance of role modelling, and that they need to be reflective practitioners or educators themselves. There is a wealth of literature focusing on the development of the reflective teacher and the facilitation of reflective learning, including, for example, Brookfield (1995), Scanlan and Chernomas (1997), Brockbank and McGill (1998), Light and Cox (2001), and Driscoll (2007).

Facilitators may prepare themselves by following the guidelines below:

- Review all exercises from a personal point of view, as well as from an educational perspective. If you have not had the opportunity to engage in the exercises as a participant prior to being a facilitator, it is recommended that you at least challenge yourself with the on-your-own exercises.
- Be prepared to role model, or participate, in all exercises. It is essential that the facilitator demonstrate an openness and willingness to share experiences. After all, this is what you are asking the group to do.

Some participants may see reflecting on experiences as uncomfortable and challenging. Facilitators can provide support and encouragement by example.

- Co-facilitation is suggested, depending upon the size of the group. With more than one facilitator, participants can benefit by the increased accessibility of a facilitator. The facilitators may also benefit from arranging to engage in ongoing dialogue and reflection with a peer.
- Bearing in mind the limitations of such a programme of exercises, and the fact that they are in no way intended to be comprehensive, facilitators should be prepared to guide participants to further appropriate resources.
- Ground rules would need to be established when working with a group in this way. These might include agreement about: listening to each other with respect, giving and being open to support, time management and keeping confidences. In our experience, these are potential pitfalls.
- Consider taking advantage of information technology where appropriate. E learning and electronic discussion boards in particular, whilst not a substitute for face-to-face communication, can be a useful resource.

Self-awareness

To be self-aware is to be conscious of one's character, including beliefs, values, qualities, strengths and limitations. It also encompasses the social self – that which others influence and shape. This will include culture, education and socialisation. Burnard (1992) distinguishes between the inner self, how one feels inside, and the outer self, the aspects that other people see, including appearance, verbal and non-verbal behaviour. Self-awareness may be described as the foundation skill upon which reflective practice is built. It underpins the entire process of reflection because it enables people to see themselves in a particular situation and honestly observe how they have influenced the situation and how the situation has affected them. Self-awareness enables a person to analyse their own feelings, beliefs and values, as a part of the social world, an essential part of the reflective process. It is evident from influential literature that it is the use of self-awareness and personal knowledge that differentiates reflective learning from other types of mental activity, for example logical thinking and problem solving (Mezirow 1981; Boud et al. 1985). All adult learners need to be self-aware in order to take responsibility for identifying and responding to their own learning needs and to consider how these impact on others. It is also important, although obvious, to state that self-awareness is essential, not only for reflective learning, but also for skilled professional nursing practice. In particular, knowledge of one's own beliefs, values and behaviour, and how these affect others is essential for developing good interpersonal skills and building therapeutic relationships with patients. In some ways, self-awareness is hard to avoid, as self-interest is part of human nature. However, developing an honest self-awareness is more complex. It is natural to want to see and portray oneself in the most favourable light. This desire, together with our own prejudices and assumptions, can sometimes interfere with the ability to take a more objective look at oneself. Being honest about oneself therefore requires courage, confidence, a certain degree of maturity and the support of others. In particular, to develop and maintain an appropriate level of self-awareness in the work situation and for reflective practice requires substantial effort and mental energy. One is sometimes dealing with deeply held values and strong feelings which may be uncomfortable and anxiety provoking. There may, therefore, be times when one chooses to avoid the process, and when it becomes more appropriate just to go home and relax. It is, however, important to bear in mind that identifying and releasing ones feelings, both positive and negative, is generally better for a person, provided that the time and place are appropriate. Whilst a degree of personal insight and self-awareness is necessary to engage in reflective practice, it is also important to recognise that too much negative introspection and analysis can have an adverse effect. Therefore, there is a need to gain the right balance in any situation.

The following series of exercises aim to help you to identify and clarify your own beliefs, values and feelings. There are also exercises enabling you to examine your motivation for developing a more reflective type of practice, and the degree to which you are open and receptive to new ideas. These factors have been identified as essential prerequisites for reflective practice (Boud *et al.* 1985; Wong *et al.* 1997).

On-your-own exercise: **Clarifying values** *15 minutes*

A personal value can be described by a statement that says what is important and significant to you as an individual in either or both of your professional and personal lives. Describe three of your own values below by completing this sentence:

It is important to me that . . .

1) . . .
2) . . .
3) . . .

> *With-a-partner exercise*: Exploring values *30 minutes*
>
> - Are you both clear and certain about what your values are? Give examples. Identify together some values that are key for you both.
> - Do your values always guide your actions? Give examples of when they have done and when they have not.
> - How did you acquire the key values in your life? Identify specific people or situations that have affected your values.
> - Compare your answers and consider how you can become clearer about your own values.

Values perform an important function for everyone. They provide a clear framework for our perspectives on life and they provide a basis for action. Being clear about your values in professional practice is also important because it will help you to live with the results of your actions. What is interesting about values is that they are chosen, but they are not necessarily consistent with one another.

> *On-your-own exercise*: How motivated am I? *15 minutes*
>
> Think about the reasons why you want to develop the skills to use reflection. Make a list of these.

You may have identified some good reasons for becoming a reflective practitioner. In addition to enabling you to develop and enhance your nursing practice, reflection is important within formal professional courses, and when profiling learning for professional registration purposes, for the assessment and accreditation of prior experiential learning (APEL) and for demonstrating work-based learning. If, however, you believe you have little to gain personally or professionally you may find it more difficult to devote the necessary time. There is always the possibility that this is not the right approach for you or that this is not the right time for you to undertake the exercises.

If you are working on these exercises alone, try teaming up with a colleague who is willing to try them out too – this may help to get you motivated.

> *On-your-own exercise*: Am I open to new ideas?
> *30 minutes*
>
> Identify from your professional practice a situation where a colleague introduced a change that would or did have implications for your own practice:
>
> Contd.

- Describe what the change was.
- What were the significant background factors to this change?
- What were your thoughts about it?
- Identify your feelings about the change.
- How receptive were you to the change? Why was this?
- What were the prejudices and biases that influenced your receptiveness?

This exercise may have highlighted two issues. First, change may not be necessarily for the better. It may be that you had negative feelings towards the change, and that this was because you did not see the change as in the best interests of the team or of the patients. It may be that you felt that there was insufficient evidence to support the change. Second, you may find change in itself difficult; if so, you need to consider carefully the reasons why you feel this way. Change can make people feel insecure and unsettled. There may also be some periods in your life when you are more receptive to change than at other times. It is, however, important to remember that an openness to new ideas is necessary to be a reflective practitioner. Working through some of the exercises will help you to develop a more positive approach to change; it can be uncomfortable and a good facilitator or supportive colleague could help.

On-your-own exercise: Your life map *15–30 minutes*

On a large piece of paper draw a map or diagram that represents the background and history of your nursing practice or training. Include as much detail as possible. Putting your nursing practice into a picture format may seem awkward or difficult at first, but it will allow you to see your career from a very different perspective. Don't worry about drawing things correctly, just try to be creative.

Include as many of the following events as possible:

- your starting point
- achievements
- joys
- sadnesses
- important people
- obstacles

With-a-partner exercise: **Directions and destinations.**
30–60 minutes

Take turns explaining the map of your career in nursing or in training. Give as much detail as possible, so that your partner can understand your background.

When listening to your partner, pay close attention to the details. Ask questions to better understand your partner's experiences. Also listen for what is left out of your partner's story.

Here are some questions you may want to use to probe a little deeper.

- Where are you on your map? How active or passive are you?
- Where are the strongest emotions on your map? What are these emotions? Have any emotionally strong experiences been left out?
- Are there any other people on your map? Who are they? Is anyone missing who should be there?
- Are there patients on your map? Why or why not?
- What takes up the most space on your map? Why do you think it does?
- Are there any empty spaces on your map? Should something else be included in those spaces? Is there any meaning in the emptiness?

Group exercise: **Looking for the crossroads.**
30–60 minutes

All participants should post their 'maps' on the walls of the room. Without describing or analysing the maps, look for what is common:

- themes
- symbols
- depictions
- colour choices
- any developments or sequences (e.g. from left to right, or bottom to top)

Given the fact that members of the group have lived through similar times and are engaged in the same profession, it is not surprising that there may be common areas. Consider how you can value the shared experiences, since they can bind the group together and also provide support. Look also for the differences between the 'maps'. These unique versions are valuable to the group in a different way in providing new perspectives. Spend a few minutes talking about the experience of 'mapping'. Allow each participant a chance to answer the question:

- What was the biggest surprise or insight you got from your own or others' life maps?

Doing life maps reminds us of the positive aspects of our careers, but it will also bring to mind the low points or sadnesses that we have experienced. Group members and facilitators should be prepared to support members of the group who need it.

Description

To describe something, whether it is a person, an object, a situation or an abstract concept or idea, is to state its characteristics or appearance without expressing a judgement. A descriptive account is usually in spoken or written form, but may also be in other forms, such as a painting or sculpture.

In appreciating the qualities and power of good description, examples of excellent descriptive accounts are widely available within English literature. In particular, the reader is referred to Styles and Moccia's (1993) anthology entitled *On Nursing – a Literary Celebration*, which contains many rich descriptive accounts of nursing and people's experiences of health and illness. Outside of nursing, the many novels of Charles Dickens contain superlative description and may provide you with an entertaining break from nursing literature.

In professional practice, good descriptive abilities are necessary when communicating verbally with colleagues about patients and for writing clear and accurate patient progress notes. When using reflection-on-action, description is the skill with which you recollect the important events and features of your practice. Good description is about giving a clear and comprehensive account of a situation. The account should include the following key elements:

- significant background factors (the context);
- the events as they unfolded in the situation;
- what you were thinking at the time;
- how you were feeling at the time;
- the outcome of the situation.

Your description should *reconstruct the situation*, to enable someone who was not there to understand the situation from your position. What you are trying to do is paint a vivid picture that then allows yourself and others to review the situation.

Some people are gifted with the skill of description, while others struggle to find the most appropriate words to express themselves. A full vocabulary is necessary to be able to describe situations, but at the same time there is a need to avoid the use of jargon and terminology which the reader or listener may not understand. It is also important to discriminate between relevant and irrelevant information. A good descriptive account, therefore, demonstrates a full and clear understanding of the relevant and important issues, and is well structured and concise.

Within a piece of written reflection, or when engaging in reflection with another person or a group, it is also important to achieve a balance between description of the situation and the analytical processes that follow. In particular, when undertaking work for academic purposes, it is often the higher-order thinking skills of analysis and evaluation that are most valued. However, it may be more difficult to engage in these critical thinking processes without good underlying descriptive skills.

On-your-own exercise: The power of description.
30 minutes

Choose a page of literature from a favourite text, for example a novel, autobiography or poem. Read it carefully. When you feel that you are really familiar with the passage, write down:

- key elements of the description that capture the essence of the situation;
- important words or phrases that facilitated your understanding.

It is important to consider what the elements of good description are. If you are able to incorporate these into your writing, you are more likely to give the comprehensive account that enables you to demonstrate your learning through experience. A good piece of description paints a vivid picture of a unique situation. It enables the reader to understand the situation from the writer's perspective. The description contains details that not only capture the significant background factors, but also bring to life these situations through the use of carefully selected words.

On-your-own exercise: 'I remember when. . . .' *30 minutes*

Identify a work situation in which you were involved recently. The situation might include one or more of the following features:

- You felt that your actions made a real difference to a patient or group of patients.

Contd.

- It went unusually well.
- It did not go as planned.
- It was very ordinary and typical of your professional practice.
- It captures the essence of what your professional practice is about.

Take some time to think about the situation. Bearing in mind the features of good description, write down as many of the details that you can remember. You need to avoid using the specific names of people or places involved, to preserve anonymity and confidentiality. Be sure to include information on the following:

- where and when the situation occurred;
- who was involved in the situation;
- the specific circumstances of the care provided/not provided;
- how you felt about the situation at the time;
- what you did at the time of the situation;
- how you coped after the situation;
- what you thought and felt about the situation at a later time.

With-a-partner exercise: 'Let me tell you about. . . .'
30–60 minutes

Using your notes from the on-your-own exercise, take it in turns to tell your partner of your experience. Don't be limited by what you wrote. Use your notes as a starting point. When listening to your partner, pay close attention to the details. Ask questions to better understand your partner's experiences. Also listen for what is left out of your partner's story. You may want to probe a little deeper. In telling this story did you talk more about what you felt, thought and did, or did you describe the actions and attitudes of others?

To facilitate another person's understanding of a situation, you need to give all the relevant factors in enough detail. A common problem may be that because you were involved in the situation, you may omit certain details that you have taken for granted. You may also find it difficult to recall the entire key factors in the situation because you have to rely on your memory. It is likely that the situations you will be most able to describe are those that occurred more recently. Sometimes it is important that you can describe situations from your nursing practice, even though they may have occurred some time ago. Keeping a diary that records and describes events in your professional practice may therefore enhance your descriptive abilities.

On-your-own exercise: Describing feelings. *30 minutes*

Think of a situation in your professional practice where the outcomes were not what you expected or you felt uncomfortable about them. Describe the situation using the elements of good description, and then answer the following questions:

- Does your description capture the essence of the situation?
- Does what you have written describe your feelings accurately and truthfully?

It is not always easy to describe the feelings you have. Some people find it easier to describe their thoughts about a situation rather than their feelings. When feelings are strong, for example, when we are very happy or very upset, they tend to be easier to acknowledge. However, in any situation there are likely to be feelings beneath the surface that may need more detailed exploration to uncover. Some people find it easier to express feelings than others. If this is true for you, you need to consider some of the reasons why this might be the case. It is, however, generally believed that we are better off identifying and releasing feelings (Boyd and Fales 1983; Brockbank and McGill 1998).

Critical analysis

Critical analysis is a key skill for both reflective practice and academic study. Analysis involves the separation of a whole into its component parts. To analyse something, whether an object, a set of ideas or a situation, is to undertake a detailed examination of the structure or constituent parts or elements and ask questions about them, in order to more fully understand their nature and how the parts relate to, and influence, each other. The term '*critical*' introduces a further dimension to analysis, in that judgements are made about the strengths and weaknesses of the different parts, as well as of the whole. Being critical does have some negative connotations when it is used in every-day life, in that it is a term often associated with finding fault. However, engaging in critical analysis, or undertaking a critique of something, is a positive and constructive process, because it is about identifying strengths as well as weaknesses. Weaknesses can be seen more helpfully as opportunities for change and to move on. Examples of using critical analysis in professional practice include assessing the needs of an individual patient, as well as making a broader contribution to service and policy development.

Some authors emphasise critical analysis as a rational, linear, problem-solving process grounded in the scientific approach (Siegel 1988; Fisher

1995). However, the more widely accepted view appears to be that critical analysis and critical thinking involve an emotional dimension (Brookfield 1987; Daly 1998; Light and Cox 2001). Acknowledging and analysing beliefs, values and feelings are a fundamental and important part of reflection if the outcome is to have a positive effect on professional learning, practice and ultimately the quality of patient care. As a health care professional, the situations you are involved in may be unique, and therefore the knowledge that you need in order to understand and solve problems in practice will depend upon the individual components of the situation and the broader context. It is also important to recognise that any situation will be influenced by your own feelings, attitudes and behaviour. When engaging in reflective practice, therefore, the skill of critical analysis involves the following activities:

- identifying and illuminating existing knowledge of relevance to the situation;
- exploring feelings about the situation and the influence of these;
- identifying and challenging any assumptions you may have made;
- imagining and exploring alternative courses of action (Brookfield 1987).

Identifying existing knowledge

The knowledge required for understanding a specific situation needs to be identified and scrutinised. You may find that in order to shed light on that situation, you need to search for and examine other knowledge that at first may not have seemed relevant. It is therefore important that you identify the types and sources of knowledge that you use in your professional nursing practice. This is about raising questions such as 'What do we know?' and 'How do we know it?'

Professional knowledge, and nursing knowledge in particular, has been classified in a number of different ways (Carper 1978, 1992; Higgs and Titchen 2000). While recognising that any classification is artificial, and different types of knowledge are interdependent, it is sometimes helpful to refer to a framework or classification when examining one's own knowledge. In Western philosophy, a common distinction has been made between propositional knowledge or 'knowing-that', which comprises theoretical knowledge, and knowledge generated through research; and non-propositional knowledge or 'knowing-how', which consists of personal knowledge, practical skills, informal knowledge and expertise (Polanyi 1958; Higgs and Titchen 2000). The work of Carper (1978, 1992) has been influential within nursing theory, and is used in some frameworks for reflection, for example, Johns (2005). Carper identifies four fundamental patterns of knowing from an analysis of the structure of nursing knowledge:

- Empirical knowledge – factual, descriptive and theoretical knowledge, often developed through research.
- Aesthetic knowledge – knowledge gained more subjectively, through unique and particular situations, and sometimes referred to as the art of nursing.
- Personal knowledge – knowledge of self, used, for example, in building therapeutic relationships with patients and in helping them cope with illness.
- Ethical knowledge – concerned with understandings and judgements of what is right, wrong or ought to be done in different situations.

Therefore, engaging in a thorough critical analysis involves analysing one's knowledge and, where necessary, actively seeking out the ideas, theories and research of others in order to look at them critically in the light of one's own knowledge.

Exploring feelings related to the situation

In reflective practice, it is necessary to gain an appropriate balance between the analysis of knowledge and the analysis of feelings. It is also important to focus on positive feelings as well as trying to deal with negative feelings, in order for the process to be constructive (Boud et al. 1985). Not only are we concerned about how our feelings affect the care we give, but to be reflective, we must also be aware of, and constructively use, our own emotions.

Identifying and challenging assumptions

Identifying assumptions is about recognising when something is taken for granted or presented as fact without supporting evidence. It is about not taking things at face value. When analysing a situation it may be helpful to ask questions like 'What is being taken for granted here?' and 'Am I representing an accurate picture of the situation?' It may be easy to carry on through our working and personal lives with the same set of assumptions, beliefs and values about oneself, about nursing and about health care practice in general. However, there is a need to challenge these assumptions regularly, and to question where they have come from. Indeed Jarvis (1992) suggests that we can easily miss crucial factors in practice by not seeing 'the extraordinary within the ordinary'; we have to see situations that we take for granted differently. Challenging the relevance of the context of nursing practice is particularly important. Events are embedded within a certain context, so it is important to be able to examine the ideas of people from different backgrounds, alongside our own. Assuming that ideas and practices that work in one context can automatically be carried to another can cause problems. Examples of such difficulties have sometimes been evident in attempts to apply

North American nursing models and health care systems to nursing in the UK.

When identifying and challenging assumptions, it is important to be sceptical of claims to universal truth. Simply because a practice has existed for a long time does not mean that it is the most appropriate. Just because an idea is accepted by others does not mean that one has to believe in its innate truth, without first checking its correspondence with one's own experience (Brookfield 1987).

Challenging the assumptions underlying one's own ideas and those of others can be an uncomfortable experience and may involve asking awkward questions. It is therefore important to raise awareness, prompt, nurture and encourage the process without making others feel threatened.

Imagining and exploring alternative courses of action

Central to this is the idea of constantly looking for new ways of thinking and new ways of doing things. Such new ways of practising allow for creativity and growth as opposed to routine and stasis. You could ask yourself the following questions: 'Do I still work in the same way as I did 2 years ago? Is that appropriate? What, if anything, do I want to do about that?' This aspect of critical analysis also requires one to look at perspectives other than one's own.

> *On-your-own exercise*: Analysing your knowledge.
> *30 minutes*
>
> Take a situation previously described. Think about the knowledge that has enabled you to understand the situation. Write a detailed account of relevant knowledge and indicate the sources of the knowledge.

Some of the knowledge you have used is likely to have been gained through personal experience. Remember that while this is a useful and valid way of gaining knowledge, you need to explore the extent to which this knowledge helps you understand the situation. Some knowledge may have been gained through 'trial and error'. It is particularly important to question this knowledge and its value. In the climate of evidence-based professional practice, formal knowledge must be a key source of understanding, and it is important that your account contains research-based knowledge where appropriate. If you have been unable to identify any formal sources of knowledge, it may be that you need to do some further thinking and reading. Group or cultural knowledge can be more difficult to identify, as this knowledge is often implicit in every-day practice. It may be taken for granted or be bound up in the assumptions that underlie your practice. It is important that you explore any assumptions you may make.

With-a-partner exercise: Discussing your knowledge.
30–60 minutes

Ask a partner to read the situation you described previously. Discuss together the knowledge that each of you considers is relevant to understanding the situation:

- Was the knowledge that your partner identified the same or different to yours?
- If different, explore the reasons why.
- Agree with your partner which knowledge is most important for understanding the situation.
- Try to identify together any new knowledge that would be relevant to the situation, and suggest alternative knowledge which may give new insights.

On-your-own exercise: Analysing your feelings. *30 minutes*

Taking a situation described previously, identify any parts that involved feelings. Read through the section carefully. See whether you have identified your feelings where appropriate. If not, why not? Try to explore honestly why you felt the way you did.

If necessary, try again to identify your feelings. Taking the relevant passage, think carefully and identify the feelings that were important in that situation. This may include feelings you had within the situation and about it, the feelings you had at the time and the feelings you have now.

Answer the following questions:

- Why did you feel the way you did?
- What are the elements that made you feel that way?
- Was there anything relevant in your past experiences that led you to feel the way you did?

With-a-partner exercise: Talking about feelings.
30 minutes

Talk through your feelings with someone you trust.

Reflective practice does involve an analysis of feelings, and without this understanding you may miss real opportunities in your experience to learn about yourself. Increasing self-awareness and the ability to analyse your feelings will give you insights that may enhance your professional practice. While analysis of feelings is difficult, if you have not been able to undertake this exercise, you need to consider carefully the reasons why.

On-your-own exercise: 'One way of looking at it.'
30 minutes

Critically analyse a situation previously described, from as many different perspectives as possible. Try to imagine the point of view of patients, colleagues and other people who were involved in the situation.

With-a-partner exercise: 'Different ways of looking at it.'
30–60 minutes

Practice taking opposing opinions on the situation presented in the previous exercise. Try defending a perspective that is not your own. Support your views with formal knowledge or theory where possible.

Frequently, health care professionals operate from substantially different viewpoints. When a dilemma presents itself, people react differently based on their beliefs and experience. The resulting conflict can be both upsetting and baffling. It may be hard sometimes to understand how equally concerned caregivers can have opposing opinions. However, in the climate of inter-professional working it is becoming increasingly important to understand and respect the values of others. Do not overlook the richness of diversity. We are open to differences in our patients and clients and need to be equally open to differences in our professional relationships.

Group exercise: The great debate. *30–90 minutes*

Divide the group into several teams, depending on the size of the group. Each team should identify and will then represent a key theory used in professional nursing practice. The teams should be asked to debate the following question:

Contd.

- What theory provides the most value to health care providers?

Team members should work together to develop their arguments. One or two members of the team should be selected as spokespersons for the group.

Round 1 – each team is allowed 5 minutes to state the reason that their theory is the most useful to health care providers.

Round 2 – each team is given 5 minutes to state the reasons why the other theories presented are inadequate in meeting the needs of health care providers.

Success of the teams will be based on the clarity of their communication and arguments.

Synthesis

Synthesis is defined by the *Oxford Dictionary* as 'the process or result of building up separate elements, especially ideas, into a connected and coherent whole'. It could be described as the opposite of analysis. Synthesis is about the artistry of professional practice, and about being creative. It often involves original thinking. At a fundamental level of practice, devising a patient care plan is an example of the synthesis of information from a variety of different sources. A good care plan is unique to the individual patient and is dynamic and changing.

When using reflection, synthesis is the ability to integrate new knowledge, feelings or attitudes with previous knowledge, feelings or attitudes. This is necessary in order to develop a fresh insight or a new perspective on a situation and therefore to learn from it. The skill of synthesis is necessary, therefore, in order to achieve a satisfactory outcome from reflection. This may include the clarification of an issue, the development of a new attitude or way of thinking about something, the resolution of a problem, a decision made or a change in behaviour. Such changes may be small or large. New knowledge may potentially be generated and original ideas or fresh ways of approaching problems or answering questions may be developed. Synthesis involves making choices with regard to relating new ideas to one's past beliefs and values. This may not be an easy process, depending upon the scope of adjustment being made. You may choose *not* to incorporate new ideas and instead maintain the existing ones; this is not necessarily right or wrong. Changing old ideas should not be done indiscriminately. The important point is that the choice is an informed decision.

The skill of synthesis can be a difficult one. Listening to the way others have put the pieces together in relation to different situations may be helpful at this point.

Chapter 2

On-your-own exercise: 'Dear Friend. . . .' 30 minutes

Take some time to think about what you have learned from the previous exercises and write a letter to a friend, real or imagined, telling of the changes you have experienced. Be sure to include some of the following:

- Give an update on yourself and your self-awareness – Has it changed? What did you learn by mapping out your career and talking it over with a partner?
- Describe one of the situations that you believe has most influenced your practice.
- Include information about the knowledge or theory you believe has most relevance to your practice.
- Finish off by writing about what you intend to do differently in identifying and handling some of the issues you encounter in your practice.

With-a-partner exercise: Spotlight on you. 30–60 minutes

In addition to the written reflections that you have undertaken during these exercises, you now have the opportunity to make an audio-visual recording. By recording your thoughts you will be able to hear and see yourself express your views about your nursing practice. You will also be able to use the recording as a yardstick against which to measure your professional growth in the future. On completion, the record will be yours alone. There will be no need to share it with anyone other than your partner for the exercises. However, you may choose to show it to a facilitator, friend, family member or mentor, or you may decide to view it again in the privacy of your own home. You have done all the preparation for this experience in the previous exercises. There is no need to use notes or check your readings. Your partner will prompt you with the questions below:

1. Tell me a little bit about who you are. (Remember the information that you put in the map of your career. You may wish to add to that information.)
2. Think of a meaningful incident in your professional career. Tell me:
   - what your role was;
   - what were the choices that you had;
   - what was the choice you made;
   - how you felt about your choice.

Contd.

(You do not need to use the incident you described previously in the section on description. Discussion of that incident may have brought to mind other situations that you have faced in practice.)

3. What type of work you would like to see yourself ultimately doing? What changes and improvements would you make in the way you approach and handle the issues that you face?

Try answering these questions in the following time frames:

- 1-year goals;
- 5-year goals;
- end of practice goals.

The idea of making an audio-visual recording of yourself may be intimidating. You may wonder if it is necessary. One of the reasons you are strongly encouraged to record yourself in this session is that it allows you the rare opportunity of seeing yourself. Unlike home movies, in which the emphasis may be on how you look, this recording will focus on what you say and how you say it. You will be able to see yourself as others see you and gain a different perspective on yourself. An audio-visual recording, unlike a written account, is more spontaneous, allowing you to say what is on your mind without worrying about punctuation or grammar.

Group exercise: The audio-visual experience.
30–90 minutes

Looking at oneself in pictures or on audio-visual records can be an unnerving experience that many approach with fear and others simply avoid. Having just created a record of yourself, it is a good time to discuss the experience. As a group, try to take a look at the benefits and risks of having been recorded. Each participant should independently write down all the advantages and all the disadvantages that the experience presents. Then, going around the room, each participant should mention one plus and one minus about the exercise that has not yet been mentioned by the other participants. Keep circling the group until all the items on everyone's list have been mentioned.

Contd.

Listing all the pluses and minuses on a flip chart will give participants a 'master list'. Reviewing this complete list will allow individuals,
as well as the group, to make a final decision on the merits of this
experience. You may find that this discussion will give you new ideas
on how you can review and use your recording in the future.

Evaluation

Evaluation is the ability to make a judgement about the value of something. It entails a 'looking back'. Judgements are often made with reference to predefined criteria or standards, for example when assessing the
value of a research report, when determining whether or not a patient
has achieved certain goals or when monitoring and auditing the extent
to which targets have been achieved within health services. Evaluation is
a high-level skill in both reflective practice and academic study. Unfortunately, the idea of evaluation can make people feel uncomfortable,
because of its association with examinations, performance appraisals and
assessment. The fear of being judged badly may make people want to
avoid it altogether.

Self-assessment or evaluation is a personal process in which one exam-
ines oneself, frequently over time. This is an important component of
reflective practice and professional education. While we can receive input
from others and include their observations and opinions, ultimately one
must judge oneself. People can frequently be their own toughest critics.
Evaluation is not meant to be self-torture for past misdemeanours. Rather
it should be *future orientated*, for example it may involve finding discrep-
ancies between what is said and needed and what is actually done, in
order to make necessary changes. Autobiographies often contain interesting examples of self-evaluation, showing how people look back on
their lives. Try reading some.

On-your-own exercise: Listening to yourself and others.
15–30 minutes

Play back your own or, with permission, your partner's audio-visual
recording. Listen to what you or your partner says on the recording
and take notes on the following:

- beliefs/values;
- problems to overcome;
- goals for the future.

With-a-partner exercise: Learning from the past and looking to the future. *30–60 minutes*

Review with your partner the notes that you have taken about the audio-visual recording. Ask your partner if he/she agrees with each of the items you have put into the categories of beliefs/values, about problems to overcome, and goals for the future.

After the discussion with your partner, change any of the items if necessary.

Use the rest of the time with your partner to identify the following:

- ongoing support systems;
- ongoing strategies;
- outlook for the next year of practice.

Group exercise: Closure. *30–90 minutes*

For the last gathering of the group, it is good to look back on the experience, look forward, and look inward at the group. This session should be a time to review and acknowledge all the hard work that went into the exercises. This last session should be personalised by the group in a way that participants feel most appropriate to their experience. A celebration might be in order!

A more wide-ranging approach to developing reflective practice

As we indicated earlier, many of the skills-based exercises in this chapter are aimed at nurses who are at the beginning of their reflective journey. However, some of you may have used earlier editions of this book, or other texts, to get started in reflection. You may now be wishing to develop your reflective practice further. For those nurses, we present some work drawn from that of Schön (1983, 1987). This work outlines some attributes or characteristics of the reflective practitioner that can be used to focus development. You may like to undertake an academic or practice-based course to help you acquire some of these characteristics, although we would suggest that they are best acquired through mentoring or coaching in practice.

Attributes of the reflective practitioner

- Demonstrating artistic practice

A reflective practitioner demonstrates what is often called an 'artistic performance', revealing knowledge in 'intelligent action' and thus showing 'knowing in action' (Schön 1987). The practitioner holds many perspectives on a practice situation, taken from a repertoire of past experiences that the professional may consider whilst in a practice situation. In situations of uncertainty, the artistic performer will reflect without interruption in his/her action (Schön 1987).

● Possessing a repertoire of experience

A reflective practitioner brings the past to bear on new situations by recalling them from a repertoire of experience – recognising similarities between previous experiences and the new one (Schön 1983). He or she has a huge range and variety of repertoire and is conscious of this when bringing it to unfamiliar situations (Schön 1983). The reflective practitioner sees the new situation as something already in his or her repertoire to an extent – seeing similarities and differences with previous experience (Schön 1983). Throughout this, the reflective practitioner will keep an open mind, and each new situation contributes to the repertoire (Schön 1983).

● Being able to frame problems and experiment in practice

Reflective practitioners will act in a new situation as they have in others, but the new problem-solving behaviour is a variation on the old – 'seeing as' they did before and 'doing as' they did before (Schön 1983). Professionals frame and re-frame problems to reshape them into an hypothesis (Schön 1983), follow rules that have not yet been made explicit and invent new rules 'on the spot' (Schön 1987). As they invent experiments to put new theories to the test, practitioners restructure the usual theories of practice (Schön 1987) and behave more like researchers than experts (Schön 1987). As the nurse experiments to discover the consequences of certain actions, the situation 'talks back' to allow re-framing of the problem (Schön 1983).

● Having an ability to articulate your reflective practice

A reflective practitioner may be limited in articulation of what she or he does by the language available (Schön 1987). The practitioner may, however, be able to articulate the new situation 'in light of' the old one (Schön 1983). Reflective practice is not, however, dependent upon being able to articulate what is done or what it reveals about a practitioner (Schön 1987). The reflective practitioner can describe deviations in practice from the norm but not what the norm is (Schön 1987). He or she can recognise a whole entity for what it is but not be immediately able to say how this recognition takes place (Schön 1987).

● Having a transactional and constructivist relationship with practice

A reflective practitioner holds a *reflective conversation* with the situation (Schön 1983). This is a transactional relationship (Schön 1983) with the unique situation as the professional waits for the results of experimentation to 'talk back'. He or she constructs situations of practice in transaction with the world of practice (Schön 1987) to construct a unique world of practice.

- Possessing tacit knowledge

The competence of reflective practice is of a high-powered, esoteric nature (Schön 1983). The practitioner demonstrates 'on-line anticipation and adjustment' in detecting and correcting errors in practice. The professional demonstrates tacit knowledge (Schön 1987) in the ways in which outcomes are anticipated and combines knowing in action and a smooth performance (Schön 1983).

I wonder how you feel after reading all this? It might be that you think that this is a very 'tall order', and it is, but many of you, particularly those who have long experience in nursing, will be already demonstrating these attributes in your daily work. Here are some thinking points that may be of help:

> ### Thinking point # 1
>
> When next in practice, stop for a moment and consider where the knowledge for your actions comes from. Think about your experience, your 'repertoire' and how you ascertain 'clues' from practice situations that suggest a certain line of action.

We can often find several sources of knowledge for practice decisions; this supports our 'world of practice'. It is unique to us as individual practitioners, but others share the same experiences. We all 'experiment' in practice to a certain degree. One of the difficulties with this is that the practice world is full of procedures and guidelines that can limit us in the actions we take.

> ### Thinking point # 2
>
> Consider an incident where you took action that differed from what would be considered to be the 'norm' for that situation. What prompted you to act differently? What was it in the situation that caused you to take this course of action? How did you know whether what you did was the best action (or not)?

We sometimes find it difficult to talk with colleagues about such situations – particularly if we have deviated from an established 'norm'. However, many of these 'norms' are unwritten rules or just constitute what is usually acceptable practice in a particular context. It can take quite a lot of courage to admit that you have done something differently. In fact, sometimes we are not totally aware that we have done so; it just comes 'instinctively'.

Thinking point # 3

To what extent is the practice knowledge that you possess derived from practice? How much comes from more formal learning? Are there differences in the type of knowledge that comes from these two sources?

This understanding of how we gain and develop our knowledge for practice is useful in that it highlights not only the amount of understanding that we derive from our daily work, but also how very important this knowledge is. It is easy, and common, for nurses to de-value this. Reflective practice is about an awareness of where our understandings come from and a purposeful use of this knowledge. Finally in this section, just to say that if much of this seems to have little meaning for you at present, or if you prefer the skills-based approach, do not worry about this. We all have our own learning preferences and it may be that the 'attributes' approach will be helpful as you gain more experience and confidence in using reflection. You might also like to look at the work of Jennifer Moon (1999) who has some interesting ideas on the features of reflective practice, which suggest some attributes or characteristics of those who might fulfil this role.

Conclusion

The intention of this chapter has been to raise awareness of the key skills and attributes that we believe underlie reflective practice, and to encourage and support professional practitioners in assessing and developing these skills and attributes. It is evident that skills for reflective practice are not discrete and separate elements, but are interrelated parts of a whole reflective process. While breaking down the process of reflective practice into constituent parts may be helpful as a strategy for learning and teaching, the challenge comes with combining and integrating the different elements. This is why we have introduced the wider-ranging notion of reflective practice as a set of attributes, a 'way of being' that may be more suitable for more experienced practitioners. It is important to remember that *genuine reflective practice can only be developed by becoming immersed in actually doing it*. This is essential for developing an approach to professional practice, or a way of thinking, whereby one constantly reviews practice in order to learn and to improve standards of care. We recommend you now to Chris Bulman's chapter (Chapter 9) where you can consider some of the practical issues involved in developing reflective skills.

Acknowledgements

This chapter draws significantly on the following unpublished work:

Atkins, S. and Murphy, K. (1993) *Developing skills for profiling learning.* An unpublished open learning package. Oxford Brookes University, Oxford.

Mackin, J. (1997) *Reflections in the mirror of experience: understanding the ethical dilemmas of nursing practice.* Unpublished doctoral dissertation and open learning package. Teachers College, Columbia University, New York.

Our sincere thanks go to Kathy Murphy and Janet Mackin for their contributions.

References

Atkins, S. and Murphy, K. (1993) Reflection: a review of the literature. *Journal of Advanced Nursing*, **18**, 1188–1192.

Bloom, B.S., Englehart, M.D., Furst, E.J., Hill, W.H. and Krathwohl, D.R. (1956) *Taxonomy of Educational Objectives, Handbook 1: Cognitive Domain.* Longman, London.

Bolton, G. (2005) *Reflective Practice: Writing and Professional Development*, 2nd edn. Paul Chapman, London.

Boud, D. (1999) Avoiding the traps: seeking good practice in the use of self assessment and reflection in professional courses. *Social Work Education*, **18** (2), 121–132.

Boud, D., Keogh, R. and Walker, D. (1985) Promoting reflection in learning: a model. In: *Reflection: Turning Experience into Learning* (eds D. Boud, R. Keogh and D. Walker), pp. 18–39. Kogan Page, London.

Boyd, E.M. and Fales, A.W. (1983) Reflective learning: key to learning from experience. *Journal of Humanistic Psychology*, **23** (2), 99–117.

Brockbank, A. and McGill, I. (1998) *Facilitating Reflective Learning in Higher Education.* Society of Research into Higher Education, London/Open University Press, London.

Brookfield, S.D. (1987) *Developing Critical Thinkers: Challenging Adults to Explore Alternative Ways of Thinking and Acting.* Open University Press, Milton Keynes.

Brookfield, S.D. (1995) *Becoming a Critically Reflective Teacher.* Jossey-Bass, San Francisco.

Bulman, C. and Schutz, S. (eds) (2004) *Reflective Practice in Nursing*, 3rd edn. Blackwell, Oxford.

Burnard, P. (1992) *Know Yourself. Self-Awareness Activities for Nurses.* Scutari Press, Harrow.

Burrows, D.E. (1995) The nurse teacher's role in the promotion of reflective practice. *Nurse Education Today*, **15**, 346–350.

Burton, A.J. (2000) Reflection: nursing's practice and education panacea? *Journal
of Advanced Nursing*, **31** (5), 1009–1017.

Carper, B.A. (1978) Fundamental patterns of knowing in nursing. *Advances in
Nursing Science – Practice Orientated Theory*, **1** (1), 13–23.

Carper, B. (1992) Philosophical inquiry in nursing: an application. In: *Philosophical
Inquiry in Nursing* (eds J.F. Kiruchi and H. Simmons). Sage, Newbury Park.

Clarke, B., James, C. and Kelly, J. (1996) Reflective practice: reviewing the issues
and refocusing the debate. *International Journal of Nursing Studies*, **33**,
171–180.

Daly, W.H. (1998) Critical thinking as an outcome of nursing education. What is
it? Why is it important to nursing practice? *Journal of Advanced Nursing*, **28**
(2), 323–331.

Driscoll, J. (ed.) (2007) *Practising Clinical Supervision: A Reflective Approach for
Healthcare Professionals*. Baillière Tindall, Elsevier, Edinburgh.

Duke, S. and Appleton, J. (2000) The use of reflection in a palliative care programme: a quantitative study of the development of reflective skills over an
academic year. *Journal of Advanced Nursing*, **32** (6), 1557–1568.

Durgahee, T. (1996) Promoting reflection in post-graduate nursing: a theoretical
model. *Nurse Education Today*, **16**, 419–426.

Durgahee, T. (1998) Facilitating reflection: from a sage on stage to a guide on
the side. *Nurse Education Today*, **18**, 419–426.

Fisher, A. (1995) *Infusing Critical Thinking into the College Curriculum*. Centre
for Research in Critical Thinking, University of East Anglia, Norwich.

Gibbs, G., Farmer, B. and Eastcott, D. (1988) *Learning by Doing. A Guide to
Teaching and Learning Methods*, pp. 46–47. FEU, Birmingham Polytechnic.

Glaze, J.E (2001) Reflection as a transforming process: student advanced nurse
practitioners' experiences of developing reflective skills as part of an MSc
programme. *Journal of Advanced Nursing*, **34** (5), 639–647.

Greenwood, J. (1998) The role of reflection in single and double loop learning.
Journal of Advanced Nursing, **27**, 1048–1053.

Hannigan, B. (2001) A discussion of the strengths and weaknesses of 'reflection'
in nursing education and practice. *Journal of Clinical Nursing*, **10**, 278–
283.

Higgs, J. and Titchen, A. (2000) Knowledge and reasoning. In: *Clinical Reasoning
in the Health Professions* (eds J. Higgs and M. Jones), 2nd edn. Butterworth
Heinemann, Oxford.

Jarvis, P. (1992) Reflective practice and nursing. *Nurse Education Today*, **12**,
174–181.

Jasper, M.A. (1999) Nurses' perceptions of the value of written reflection. *Nurse
Education Today*, **19**, 452–463.

Johns, C. (2000) *Becoming a Reflective Practitioner*. Blackwell Science, Oxford.

Johns, C. (2005) *Guided Reflection*. Blackwell, Oxford.

Johns, C. and Freshwater, D. (eds) (2005) *Transforming Nursing Through Reflective Practice*, 2nd edn. Blackwell Publishing, Oxford.

Kim, H.S. (1999) Critical reflective inquiry for knowledge development in nursing
practice. *Journal of Advanced Nursing*, **29** (5), 1205–1212.

Light, G. and Cox, R. (2001) *Learning and Teaching in Higher Education: The Reflective Professional*. Paul Chapman, London.

McGill, I. and Beaty, L. (2001) *Action Learning: A Guide for Professional, Management and Educational Development*, 2nd edn. Kogan Page, London.

Mezirow, J. (1981) A critical theory of adult learning and education. *Adult Education*, **32** (1), 3–24.

Moon, J. (1999) *Reflection in Learning and Professional Development. Theory and Practice*. Routledge Falmer, Abingdon.

Page, S. and Meerabeau, L. (2000) Achieving change through reflective practice: closing the loop. *Nurse Education Today*, **20**, 365–372.

Paget, T. (2001) Reflective practice and clinical outcomes: practitioners' views on how reflective practice has influenced their clinical practice. *Journal of Clinical Nursing*, **10**, 204–214.

Paterson, B.L. (1995) Developing and maintaining reflection in clinical journals. *Nurse Education Today*, **15**, 211–220.

Polanyi, M. (1958) *Personal Knowledge: Towards a Post-Critical Philosophy*. Routledge and Kegan Paul, London.

Scanlan, J.M. and Chernomas, W.M. (1997) Developing the reflective teacher. *Journal of Advanced Nursing*, **25**, 1138–1143.

Schön, D. (1983) *The Reflective Practitioner*, 2nd edn. Jossey Bass, San Francisco.

Schön, D. (1987) *Educating the Reflective Practitioner*. Jossey Bass, San Francisco.

Siegel, H. (1988) *Educating Reason: Rationality, Critical Thinking and Education*. Routledge, London.

Styles, M.M. and Moccia, P. (eds) (1993) *On Nursing: A Literary Celebration*. National League for Nursing, New York.

Wong, F., Loke, A., Wong, M., Tse, H., Kan, E. and Kember, D. (1997) An action research study into the development of nurses as reflective practitioners. *Journal of Nursing Education*, **36** (10), 476–481.

Chapter 3

Assessing and evaluating reflection

Sue Schutz

Introduction

In this chapter, I want to turn your attention to the more structured aspects of reflection – the role of assessment and of evaluation. Reflection, as part of academic or professional courses, is often used as a learning and teaching strategy, and as a key professional skill. As an informal activity, outside of a classroom, reflection may also be used as a means of facilitating the development of new skills in practice. In both situations, assessment could be said to be valuable in order to evaluate achievements. Reflection may be a means to an end or an end in itself, but in both cases, some evaluation is needed of the success of the venture. This chapter is written for two groups of readers: (1) those who are starting out or engaged in reflection and who need to consider the role of assessment and evaluation of reflection for their own needs; and (2) those who facilitate or mentor/coach reflection in an informal or academic setting and need to make assessments of students' abilities.

Sumison and Fleet (1996) stated that little is known about how reflection and reflective practice are best promoted or measured. The body of evidence on reflection has continued to grow since the last edition of this book; however, the assessment and evaluation of reflection remain a contentious area. The aims of this chapter are to:

● define the meanings of assessment and evaluation of reflection in nursing and explore the practical and theoretical issues that this raises;
● outline and debate the existing evidence base for the assessment and evaluation of reflection.

The lack of clarity about the process of assessing reflection can be seen as an obstacle in its promotion (Newell 1994) and this poses difficulties for the assessment and evaluation of reflection. The current emphasis in health care on evidence-based practice makes this lack of evidence a pertinent issue and many authors raise this (Greenwood 1998; Burnard 1995; Johns 1995; Wallace 1996; Mallik 1998; Paget 2001). Evidence, standards and targets are a huge pressure on health and social care professionals at present and can often be perceived as being counter forces to reflective practice. However, educationalists suggest the need to *marry* organisational goals with goals for reflection (Zeichner and Liston 1987; Korthagen and Wubbels 1995), so the two are not mutually exclusive. Definitions of reflection will inevitably differ depending on the social factors influencing the development of organisations and collabo-rating practice areas, but reflective and organisational goals can comple-ment each other; after all, the espoused aims are the same.

Definitions

Discussion about definitions of assessment and evaluation of reflection may begin with the debate about what reflection actually is. However, in Chapter 1 we drew on the work of Wittgenstein in making the point that in reality some things are hard to define and so a unanimously agreed definition for reflection may be difficult. The key thing is to pay more attention to how the meaning of reflection is identified within nursing and thus develop more of an appreciation of the similarities and differ-ences in interpretations (Wittgenstein 1967). This means doing a lot more sharing between institutions on how we are tackling assessment and evaluation of reflection, and of course it means doing more research.

In addition, Sue Atkins and Sue Schutz present in Chapter 2 some putative attributes of reflective practice that may help educators to make more sound assessment of the achievement of reflection. Moreover, you may like to have a look at the work of Korthagen and Wubbels (1995) who reported on a programme of research exploring the mathematics department of a teacher education college in the Netherlands, where the fundamental goal of the programme was the promotion of reflective teaching. They define reflection from the cognitive perspective as a mental process for the structuring or restructuring of an experience, problem or existing knowledge and insights. They indicate the impor-tance of relating this to views about good teaching, which they capture through their research as having a good command of the subject but also the importance of nurturing good interpersonal relationships with stu-dents and an awareness of one's own functioning as a teacher. Thus facilitation, focusing on real and concrete problems, problem solving and learning how to learn were all key values in the programme teachers' views of good teaching. Their acknowledgment of the need to consider the link between concepts of reflective practice and good teaching is a valuable pointer in exploring the development of reflective practice in nursing, since I would suggest that practitioners' concepts of reflection will undoubtedly arise from their beliefs about good nursing.

From the summary of their research they suggest a series of critical attributes and correlates of reflection based on their explicit views of good teaching and reflection:

- Attributes
  - The reflective teacher is capable of structuring situations and problems and considers it important to do so.
  - The reflective teacher uses certain standard questions when structuring experiences such as: What happened? Why did it happen? What did I do wrong? What could I have done differently?
  - The reflective teacher can easily answer the question of what he or she wants to learn. She/he is less dependent on educators when it comes to choosing learning goals.
  - The reflective teacher can adequately describe and analyse his or her own functioning in interpersonal relationships with others.

- Correlates
  - Reflective teachers have better interpersonal relationships with students than other teachers.
  - Reflective teachers develop a high degree of job satisfaction.
  - Reflective teachers also consider it important for their students to learn by investigating and structuring things themselves.
  - Reflective teachers have previously been encouraged to structure their experiences and problems.
  - Reflective teachers have strong feelings of personal security and self-efficacy.
  - Teachers with teaching experience, who have a high degree of self-efficacy, focus, in their reflections about their teaching, on their students. When they have a low sense of self-efficacy they focus on themselves.
  - Reflective teachers appear to talk or write relatively easily about their experiences.

If you are a teacher or facilitator of reflection, I think you will find this very illuminating. It has a high degree of face validity. At this stage it is important to be clear about the terminology that we are using. The terms assessment and evaluation are sometimes used interchangeably and, in the context in which I am going to explore these activities, to continue to use them in this way would be confusing. Burnard (1988) distinguishes between the two in the context of reflective journal writing. He states that to assess is to:

> '. . . identify a particular state at a particular time, usually with a view to taking action to change or modify that state' (p.105)

and that evaluation is to:

'. . . place a value on a course of action, to identify the success or otherwise of a course of action' (p.105)

With this in mind, we can see that to assess reflection and to evaluate it are two rather different activities. Indeed, they have different aims, processes and structures. The assessment of reflection may involve a different group of people to those involved in evaluation and the timing is likely to vary. Commonly, when the assessment of reflection is raised, this refers to the ways in which students undertaking educational activities are tested in their ability to reflect on their own and others' practice. It embraces the process of reflection, the possession of the skills for reflection and the outcomes of reflection in terms of practice change. An example of this would be the assessment of an adult nursing student's written reflection on her own practice, which is contained within a learning contract. The assessor uses specific tools in order to make a judgment about the level of reflection achieved.

When the subject of evaluation of reflection is raised, I will be referring to activities that aim to uncover the value of reflection in the educational curriculum, or in nursing practice. An example of this might be the annual review of a nursing degree programme by the higher education organisation, which asks the programme team to undertake a review of the use of reflection in that course.

The assessment of reflection

Many aspects of nursing practice and education have an impact on the assessment of reflection: in particular, the setting in which students are currently engaged in practice. This may be within an institution or in the community, but it is always within the broad framework of health and social care. The complexities of the health service are familiar to us all, but it is worth spending some time exploring what it is about a health or social care setting that has an impact on reflective practice and its assessment.

The health care context

This encompasses the health care organisation as a whole and the quality of leadership and management within that organisation. Constant change within health and social care is a fact of life and it is generally recognised that this perpetual motion is due to the impact of political, technological and sociological drivers. In nursing, the situational or contextual setting of practice is of paramount importance and reflection can play a key part in helping the student to connect with the realities of practice. Students need to be equipped with the necessary skills that will help them learn from what they see and experience; the influence of the context can be very powerful. Staff in practice who are supervising students in reflective practice are also affected by these changes. The availability of quality, motivated mentors for students may be compromised, despite service/ education agreements, and learning opportunities thus impinged upon.

At many universities, factors such as these have contributed to the continual review and development of programmes to prepare nurses and other health care professionals for first-level and advanced practice. In particular, it has led to the development of changes in relation to the assessment of reflection through academic work and the use of innovative tools such as portfolios to map student development. Additionally, increased interest in the dialogic approach to reflection is noted with more and more higher education institutes introducing reflective groups and action learning sets to the nursing curriculum.

Issues in assessing reflection

The great debate in the literature is about whether reflection should actually be assessed at all or whether it is a contradiction in terms to make judgments about what is a rather personal process. This goes to the heart of the role that reflection plays in the development of the skills needed for practice. If reflection is a key skill in achieving the learning outcomes of particular courses and is acknowledged to have a positive impact on care, then it must be assessed. The literature describes the assessment of reflection in both summative ways (for example, Morgan and Johns 2005) and formative ways (as in Getliffe 1996, among others); the tensions are about both assessment of reflection per se and about the tools used if assessment is to be made.

Rich and Parker (1995) discussed the potential for what they call psychological burn when adding assessment to the (possibly painful) process of reflection. This suggests that there may be actual or potential harm in attempting to make judgments about students' abilities to reflect and adds an imperative to the debate about whether it is done at all, and if it is, how to do it 'safely'. Indeed, Cotton (2001) goes further in likening reflection to the confessional, where someone else knows one's innermost thoughts, and where one may be judged by another.

These are concerns to be taken seriously, but the fact remains that nurses (and other professionals) value professional knowledge using concepts such as reflection because they recognise the problem of the theory–practice gap and are struggling to do something about it. If nurse education does not work at ways to assess and evaluate reflection successfully, propositional knowledge will continue to dominate as the only legitimate form of knowledge in higher education. The value of informal or culturally specific knowledge can be enhanced and made legitimate through its use in practice (Eraut 1994) and through reflection. Whilst some of this informal knowledge can have a personal investment, good facilitation can help people to stay in charge of what they reveal in their verbal reflection.

There is a dilemma here in what is wanted for the purposes of assessment; is it the spontaneous, immediate response to a practice event or is it the considered reaction of later? Both are reflective. What needs to be considered is the emotional element of reflection. If time could be thought to remove or alter this, then timely reflection is most important, as emotions are a valid aspect of reflection. Some students find it useful to go back to a diary and use the benefit of hindsight to edit their reflection for the purposes of assessment. Thus they may not be writing spontaneously when being assessed, but they are able to make use of verbal, more immediate reflection with colleagues and mentors at the time and then write at a later date.

The work undertaken by Ashford et al. (1998) found that students were freer to 'take risks' (p.14) in reflection when no formal assessment is taking place. This would suggest that a more meaningful level of reflection might be possible where no judgment is going to be made. However, when reflection is used formally in courses to develop practice, some type of assessment needs to be made in order to best utilise and to map that progress; it is difficult to see how this can be omitted. This is where the use of formative as well as summative strategies is helpful. Chapter 7 by Melanie Jasper discusses the use of reflective journals and highlights the fact that not all of what is written in a reflective journal or diary may be used for formal assessment purposes. Therefore, the structure of the assessment of reflection needs to be formulated in such a way that there is opportunity for students to have both a private and a public 'version' of their reflective thoughts.

It should not, however, be assumed that the assessment of reflection in students is a kind of 'necessary evil'; Paget (2001) found that the impact of reflection on practice seemed to be enhanced by summative assessment, possibly because it is a motivator to effective reflection. However, it could just be a motivator for students to get something written even if of little meaning, so we need to be careful about putting too much pressure on students to come up with a product. Another key question that arises here is that of the clarity about what is actually being assessed; both Goodman (1984) and Mezirow (1991) assert that there are levels of reflection and therefore, without formal assessment, the level (or depth) to which an individual student is able to reflect on practice cannot be known. With the increasing use of reflective groups in education, which focus on dialogue rather than writing, reflection can be assessed verbally. (See Pam Sharp and Charlotte Maddison's discussion (Chapter 4) for some examples of how this can be done.)

It is important that educators and practitioners are clear about the outcomes of the effort put into reflection. Clearly, it is a time-consuming activity and one that carries with it an element of risk for those involved. Ghaye and Lillyman (2000) asserted that reflection must have a tangible outcome and this is difficult to measure without some form of assessment of students. This brings me to the second issue, which is how reflection might be best assessed. I noted earlier that the notion of 'private' and 'public' versions of reflective writing might be a possible answer; Hannigan (2001) sees assessment of reflection as one part of a comprehensive assessment strategy and asserts that it is how it is done that is the key. The same author advocates attention to the preparation of assessors and to the support of students and staff during the process.

In summary, where reflection is a key part of the curriculum, it needs to be assessed formally. However, the strategy used to achieve this must include both summative and formative elements, and be framed by a support system for students and assessors.

Problems with the assessment of reflection

The problem areas associated with assessing reflection are many and varied, as might be expected. The wide interpretations of what constitutes reflection and how it is practically applied make for a minefield of difficulties. The key issues that arise are listed below:

- clarifying as an organisation what constitutes reflection;
- whether it is the process of reflection or its outcome that should be assessed;
- whether reflection has levels and how these develop over time;
- barriers to honesty caused by summative assessment;
- a lack of effective tools for assessment;
- the skills of facilitators;
- political and financial pressures.

I will briefly consider each of these problem areas in turn.

Lack of clarity about what constitutes reflection

The varied interpretations of what constitutes good reflection are a problem in that students need to know what is expected of them and assessors need to know what they are looking for. However, there is an overlap in terms such as reflection, reflective practice, reflective learning, critical thinking and critical analysis (Daly 1998). Some of these are used interchangeably and some are aspects of others. Many of the skills needed for reflection, such as self-awareness and analysis, are required by more than one of these concepts. Some of the expected outcomes are also common – the improvement of practice and professional development, for example. What is important is that educational teams have a clear idea of what they mean by reflection, that this is *based on the best available evidence* and that this is *passed on to students using it*. The putative attributes of reflective practice, outlined in Chapter 2, may be of some assistance, but it is probably best not to confuse reflection and reflective practice at this point.

The process of reflection or the outcome – what should be assessed?

Burton (2000) questions whether written reflective accounts accurately demonstrate learning and development or are merely 'a perfunctory exercise to comply with . . . requirements' (p.105). This raises the question of what is actually being assessed, the process of reflecting or the impact that this has on the individual (Burns 1994; Mountford and Rogers 1996). There is no doubt that those students who possess good academic writing skills are at an advantage when written reflection is being assessed, and that there is a danger that students write what they think the assessor wants to hear (Mackintosh 1998; Platzer *et al.* 2000). This echoes Hannigan's (2001) call for comprehensive assessment strategies, which take account of this by adopting a variety of testing strategies. What is desirable is for students to engage fruitfully in reflective practice – not for them to jump through hoops. Therefore, it is both the process and the outcome that are being assessed, because they are both of equal importance. Being clear about the stages of the process of reflection and what the outcomes are is central to curriculum design (Mezirow 1991; James and Clark 1994; Lowe and Kerr 1998).

Whether reflection has levels and how these develop over time

The assessment of reflection needs to take into account the speed at which students develop these skills over time. Reflection is a complex activity and those new to reflection may have difficulty with it (Heath 1998). Indeed, it is clear that some are more naturally reflective than others and many students struggle with reflective practice for a long time. Glaze (2002) found that, in the early stages of learning to reflect, a lack of insight acted as a barrier to reflective development, and assessment during these early stages needs to take this into account. In postgraduate courses and for mature students, this is sometimes not the case because these students are often more experienced and confident people and individual evaluation of where the student 'starts at' may be needed. Burrows (1995) suggested that those under 25 years of age might lack the cognitive readiness and experience for reflective practice. This includes many undergraduate nursing students. However, this work focuses on cognition, whereas reflection is the intermingling of 'thinking', feeling and action; perhaps studies focusing on this mix may reveal a different perspective. What is important is that an assessor looks for a rounded sense of the student's reflective ability, not simply a sum of the criteria used to assess this.

Barriers to honesty caused by summative assessment

As a highly personal exercise, it is clear that bringing personal feelings and judgments into the public domain may act as a barrier to reflection. Richardson (1995) and Bolton (2005) maintained that assessment undermines effective reflection and that honesty will be compromised. In my experience, this is often the case, but other forms of reflection may offer the student an opportunity to reflect more openly and find ways of including this in assessed work without feeling exposed. The use of individual tutorials, reflective groups, action learning circles and personal diaries can all give students the chance to 'try it out' in a safe environment and, hopefully, come to terms with a level of candour that feels comfortable and aids effective reflection. Mentors and clinical supervisors also have a key role to play in encouraging and challenging reflection with their students; this is, of course, dependent on a positive relationship where trust and communication is fostered. Facilitators could also try some of the exercises presented in Chapter 2 with groups so that they may experience different approaches.

Lack of effective tools for assessment

The range of tools available for the summative assessment of reflection includes journals, learning contracts, critical incident analysis and reflective essays. For formative assessment, action learning circles, group and individual tutorials may be used. One of the problems that can arise with these methods is a lack of clarity about what is being assessed; it is important to have criteria that reflect the skills and activities necessary for effective reflection and to build in room for development over time. On postgraduate programmes, where educators are working with more experienced practitioners, problems can still arise. As Hannigan (2001) pointed out, these people are often experts in their area and use an embedded or tacit form of knowledge and thus can find it difficult to articulate what they do. Reflection can be, and often is, found by these students to be a way of articulating and making more concrete this informal knowledge. Additionally, attending seminars on reflection does not necessarily equip practitioners to do it (Paget 2001); participation in the process is what is important.

   Tools designed to assess reflection need to be flexible enough to allow students to progress at their own speed and to demonstrate their abilities to reflect in a variety of ways. Burton (2000) points out that coercion may defeat the purpose of the exercise and lead to de-motivation. Anxiety and poor memory (Andrews *et al.* 1998; Reece-Jones 1995) can all adversely affect performance, and tools to assess reflection need to allow students to perform to the best of their ability despite these barriers. For example, Burnard (1988) found that reflective diaries, which are not completed regularly, cause problems with recall and this can hinder the experience.

Skills of facilitators

The role of the facilitator of reflective learning is crucial and can make or break a reflective experience. The role of facilitator may be fulfilled by a lecturer, link lecturer, lecturer practitioner, practice teacher and/or mentor, supervisor, colleague or manager and requires very specific skills. A facilitator might not be the assessor of reflective ability and in fact this may 'muddy the waters' if he/she is. A programme of training and on-going development for those who assess reflection is important, and this needs to be well resourced. Facilitators need to have some experience of reflection and be able to offer students a balance of support and challenge. They also need to have expertise in the student's field of practice so that they can understand contextual issues that influence student experiences.

Some helpful material related specifically to facilitation skills and assessing reflection may be found in Andrews *et al.* (1998) and Durgahee (1998). The role of the facilitator in balancing the dual imperatives of facilitating and assessing may be aided by a stronger focus on formative assessment rather than the more traditional summative or final assessment. Facilitators reading this chapter will find help in other parts of this book, particularly Chapters 4, 5 and 6. There are some specifics to the role of facilitator that are worth mentioning; these may include equity in a group, time keeping, inclusion, learning approaches and others.

Political and financial pressures

The never-ending financial and resource pressures placed upon nurses can often be seen to impact negatively on our ability to effectively assess reflection in students and others. It is without doubt a time-consuming activity that in a busy care environment can be relegated to last on the list of priorities. This may be due to many factors, some of which are not directly related to real pressures. Fears in clinical staff about facilitating reflection can result in excuses about time pressures and educators need to be sure that those asked to facilitate are adequately prepared and supported. Anxiety is created through the conflicting needs of patient care, students' expectations and the demands of managers and administrators.

In the absence of a clear evidence base for reflective practice, it is often not afforded the time that it might be due. More research is needed that could indicate the potential benefits of reflection for patient care, and for service delivery in general. However, it would be hard to disagree with the notion of equipping nurses with critical thinking skills. Equipping them with reflective skills simply takes this a few steps further, since not only are we supporting and challenging students to develop their critical thinking but also we are concerned with facilitating them to develop their critical self-awareness and motivation to positively challenge and change practice, ultimately for the benefit of clients.

Tools for assessing reflection

A number of tools are available to assess students' reflective abilities and it is likely that an educational curriculum will utilise a range of these as each has strengths in the assessment of aspects of reflection. Many of these are also suitable for use in an informal setting, where reflection may be assessed as part of professional development, perhaps for clinical supervision or appraisal purposes too. The variety of tools can be divided into verbal and written strategies:

- Verbal strategies:
  - individual discussion with mentors (see Chapter 4);
  - individual and group reflective tutorials;

- Written strategies:
  - reflective learning contract;
  - critical incident analysis;
  - reflective essay;
  - reflective journal or diary;
  - reflective case studies;
  - reflective portfolio.

Each of these has its own distinct process and form; I will say a few words about each in turn, evaluating particular strengths and problem areas. Each will use the terms that are appropriate to reflection in an institute of higher education, but can be appropriate for informal assessment of reflection too, if you are using reflection as part of clinical supervision, for example. For those of you who are starting out or are engaged in reflection, the guidance given here and the points raised will give you some help in going about reflection when assessment is part of the journey.

Verbal assessment strategies

Individual discussion with mentors

The concept of reflective dialogue has been the subject of research (e.g. Phillips *et al.* 2000) and can be planned and structured or spontaneous and timely to the event discussed. Reflective discussion between mentors and students often falls into the unplanned category, and is usually timely to the event, taking place in the context of the event. I have mentioned the advantages of the former but not the impact of reflection in the setting of care. The influence of this is unknown, but one would suspect that it might help or hinder the openness of the discussion, dependent upon the particular situation. Mentors may need to be sensitive to this, and the spontaneity of the discussion may be affected by the need to find a comfortable and safe place to reflect. These kinds of reflective encounters may not be directly assessed, but they frequently feed into the assessment process. One of the mentor's responsibilities is often to validate competence in certain areas and this is likely to include reflective discussion of related events.

Students will also be developing their thinking and self-awareness in the context of real-life practice and thus such reflective discussion is likely to be used in the development of assessed written work. The preparation of mentors is key to the success of this strategy and the exploration of reflection should feature in the education of mentors. The work of Gibbs et al. (1988) and Johns (2005) is often used, I find, and may be frameworks that mentors are familiar with. Mentors work along-side students on a day-to-day basis and are familiar with the experiences that a student is exposed to. Factors such as workload, the skills of the mentor, and the culture and characteristics of the care setting will influence both the frequency of these discussions and their quality. Their success depends heavily on the mentor's confidence in making explicit his or her own thought processes and openness to challenge and debate. Work carried out by Schutz et al. (1996) showed how students perceive the relative success of a placement as depending heavily on the quality of their relationship with their mentor, and thus such qualities directly influence the level of reflective discussion. In Chapter 4, Pam Sharp and Charlotte Maddison discuss many of these points in more detail.

Individual and group tutorials

Individual and group tutorials are a regular feature of programmes for the preparation of nurses. Yet as resources become stretched, there has been pressure in many universities to minimise one-to-one tutorials, in favour of groups. The reflective tutorial can be used to focus on specific events in one student's life or to address more general issues in practice. Very often, a skilled facilitator can achieve both. The individual tutorial may be used to discuss areas that are problematic to a certain student and therefore not appropriate for groups, whilst group tutorials allow students to participate at the level at which they feel comfortable and to learn from each other. Facilitators of group tutorials need to ensure that students who are reluctant to contribute are not neglected and are able to engage as much as possible with other reflective activities in which they feel more comfortable. A good knowledge of group dynamics and well-developed skills in facilitation are very important, as students need to be in a safe and comfortable environment whilst subjects that may be challenging are debated. Heath (1998) suggested that mixing together in a group students who are at different stages of a course (and therefore likely to be at a variety of levels of reflective ability) is of benefit.

The role of reflective tutorials in the assessment of reflection is likely to be of a formative nature – allowing students to explore and develop ideas and to gain feedback on these. Research has been reported on reflective practice groups (Ashford et al. 1998) and it has been suggested that group tutorials have particular influence on students' development. In Chapter 6, the pros and cons of group reflection are debated in more depth. In many universities, teaching staff have introduced a reflective tutorial group into the curriculum, whereby students meet regularly in the group throughout the period of an undergraduate pre-registration programme. The skills needed for reflection are introduced gradually, starting with the skills of self-awareness and moving through those of description, critical analysis and evaluation. This staged approach is mindful of the concerns expressed by Heath (1998) about how novices can be overwhelmed by the new experiences to which they are exposed.

Written assessment strategies

Before discussing some of the approaches that can be used to assess reflection in a written format, it is appropriate to explore some of the issues associated with this form of assessment. In general, it is acknowledged in educational circles that some students 'take to' academic writing more easily than others. This is particularly pertinent in reflective writing because the ability to express oneself clearly and concisely is a skill that is particularly important in written reflection; Wong et al. (1995) recognised that students' writing may not be indicative of their actual reflective abilities. Reflection is a skill that does not easily lend itself to quantifiable research methods and the correlation between written and actual reflective ability remains unknown. The beauty of reflective writing is that it enables the student to relate every-day practice to theoretical learning and to enhance the reflective cycle in so doing. Being reflective embraces both verbal and written approaches.

The reflective learning contract

The reflective learning contract has been used extensively to facilitate learning directly from practice. Very often, teachers have found that the learning contract can be the 'public face' of a student's private reflective journal, and this has its drawbacks. Students have found that they cannot distinguish relevant from irrelevant material, find it difficult to include the aspect of reflection that they feel they should include, and become rather introspective (Schutz et al. 1996). Bolton (2005) proposed that formally assessed learning contracts lead to students following 'rules' of how to do it and also inappropriate levels of disclosure. She highlighted the important challenge of encouraging students to draw upon their journals or diaries rather than divulging raw reflection. The consequence of this is that students concentrate on the descriptive and emotional aspects of events to the detriment of the evaluative (Rolfe et al. 2001). The challenge for the educator is how to move students on to a higher level of reflection, and, as Fund et al. (2002) found, this is about moving to a more deliberate form of reflection, which Fund and colleagues term 'critical bridging' (p.491). At its most effective, students use the learning contract as a dialogue with the mentor and write in it regularly, asking the mentor for written feedback. (See Chapter 4 for a detailed account of this.) As a format for demonstrating reflective growth, the learning contract cannot be beaten for documenting practice-based reflection. At worst, it is time-consuming and cumbersome. Subsequently pressures related to resources, principally the precious time of qualified nursing staff, can impact negatively on the practical use of the learning contract, particularly for pre-registration undergraduate students.

Critical incident analysis

The notion of critical incident analysis is not new; it was used initially by pilots who analysed flying missions with the intent of improving their performance (Flannigan et al. 1954). Since then, Smith and Russell (1991), Norman et al. (1992) and Perry (1997) have described critical incident analysis as an appropriate strategy in nursing. The technique enables students to utilise a real event from practice that they can recall as having an impact on them. This may be a positive or negative impact. The event may be discrete, with a clear beginning and end, or more general with a variety of issues arising (Norman et al. 1992). When using this approach, I have found that it is important to give students guidance on the form that it might take. Smith and Russell (1991) provide a useful framework, which I have slightly adapted:

1. Give a concise description of the incident, highlighting the major events.
2. Outline why you chose the event and how and why it is significant to you in both personal and professional terms.
3. Identify the key issues and why they are important.
4. Reflect on:
   - how you were involved, what you felt about the events, your part in them and why;
   - why you behaved the way you did and how you made your decisions;

○ the part that others played and why you think they behaved as they did;

○ what else was happening in the context at the time and any influential circumstances;

○ the relevant theoretical background – how were events informed by theory of any type? What role did formal and informal theory play in the decisions made?

○ what action might be indicated either now or in the future;

○ how you evaluate what happened in terms of what you have learned in a specific and in a general sense.

The specific benefits of such a tool are that it can have quite formalised guidelines, allowing students to relate the practical to the theoretical and recognise the context of the situation. These factors can help the novice and also allows the experienced reflective practitioner to create more depth in reflection.

The reflective essay

The traditional essay as an assessment form is easily recognised. Such well-developed approaches can be modified effectively to assess reflective learning. The basic structure of the essay remains the same, but students are asked to write from a more personal standpoint, writing in the first person. This makes the student's own involvement explicit and allows exploration of practice using a reflective framework. An example of the title for a reflective essay might be: *Reflect on and analyse the nurse's role in discharge planning in a multi-professional setting.*

When marking a reflective essay, some of the usual 'rules' of academic writing need to be put aside. I have already mentioned that it would be written in the first person. Also the assessor would be looking for evidence of personal and professional growth; this may mean that students need to include personal thought and self-disclosure. The basic academic rules remain, such as structure, referencing and critique, but there are subtle differences. Grading criteria used to assess such work would need to embrace the reflective element and give due credit for it. This is where levels of reflection can be useful; by aligning these with grading criteria, teachers can be more specific about what is wanted at each stage and engender a developmental approach to assessing reflection.

The reflective journal or diary

Using a reflective journal is, as Melanie Jasper points out in Chapter 7, a good starting point in reflective practice. Keeping a diary preserves regular time and space for reflection in a busy life (Wong *et al.* 1995). By writing about our practice experience, we can more readily articulate the subtleties of what we do, and this is a valuable skill. The notion of

Chapter 3

assessing students' reflective diaries, however, is a problematic one. If assessment is to be used, then students need to be aware of the purpose from the outset. Richardson and Maltby (1995) used Powell's framework (1989) to explore the use of assessed diaries; they found (as Powell herself did) that the majority of students found the assessment to be a barrier to use of the diary. The danger here is that students resort to keeping a personal version of their diary and write up another for assessment; this, as Jasper points out, is a reasonable line of action, but makes the aim of assessing a diary rather pointless, because the nature of the document is subtly different.

One of the difficulties in assessing diaries or journals is the very individuality of these; grading criteria would be very difficult to construct and utilise unless this too is individual, as Burnard (1988) suggested. Additionally, equity in marking would be a real issue. If reflective diaries are used at all for assessment purposes, it is beneficial to keep the assessment very simple. Wong et al. (1995) used three grades: *reflector, non-reflector* and *critical reflector*. Students' reflective journals should be private, unless the student chooses to share the content at a tutorial, group meeting or in written work; importantly, this is entirely their choice. In this way, a reflective diary is an essential part of the assessment of reflection, but is not the actual vehicle for it. However, as a resource the diary is invaluable.

Kember et al. (2001) suggested that students are so highly assessment-driven that to remove journals from the assessment process means that they are unlikely to be kept. In my experience, it is often clear whether students use a diary, because the very act of writing a diary as the first stage in reflecting on an incident helps to sort out the relevant detail from the irrelevant. Therefore, students who keep a reflective diary and use it on which to base assessed work are likely to achieve a higher level of reflection.

Kember et al. (2001) advocated the acquisition of feedback on reflective journal entries, but this does not need to be assessed. It could be an informal arrangement between students, with a personal tutor, colleague or mentor, and still be as effective, without the burden of achieving certain criteria for assessment. Making this slightly more formal arrangement, as Kember et al. suggested, may be a useful approach, but may not be so very far from formal assessment in the students' eyes. It is vital that teachers indicate to students where the assessment points are and the nature of the assessment to be carried out.

Reflective case studies

Reflective case studies are useful in allowing students to have a go at reflection, within a structured format. Often, an additional framework is used, such as a nursing model. An assignment utilising this approach might ask a student to: *Choose one aspect of care, explore the evidence* base for practice and critically analyse the nursing management for that aspect of care. Reflect on how the nursing management of the problem could be improved.

This type of assessment enables the student to make meaningful connections between real-life practice and theoretical material. It also allows a personal approach, such that students can explore their own practice, as well as that of others. It would usually take the form of an academic piece of writing, although more creative and inclusive strategies could be used to present the case study, such as a presentation or poster. Being practice based, other forms of knowledge could be included to enable students to reflect on the array of sources from which they may draw for practice, whilst reflecting on the value of each.

The reflective portfolio

Portfolios are a statutory requirement for nurses and, for this reason, seem to be a useful way of assessing reflection in the long term. There is considerable and growing support for the use of reflective portfolios in education and this has become a popular strategy in nursing courses. The portfolio would be a collection of evidence and reflection on that evidence, to demonstrate progression in reflection over time. The advantages of the use of a portfolio to assess reflection are that:

- It can incorporate evidence of many different forms of reflection – individual, group, written and verbal.
- It is self-directed – a key skill for reflection.
- It can be built upon over time – indeed it is based on this premise;
- It allows students to work at their own reflective level.

However, there are some issues in using portfolios to assess reflection and these include the relative advantage that some students with certain learning styles may have (this is a common issue with assessment in general), the time-consuming nature of the work involved in gathering evidence and the prescriptive form that portfolios can take.

Grading reflection

Although levels of reflection are widely covered in the literature in relation to depth or progression, the association of these levels with assessment has not been further explored. It does appear that in many of these descriptors of progression in reflection, higher-level reflection embraces broader issues than just what is happening immediately around the student, to include application of theory to practice and a change in the student's perspective. Mezirow (1981) generated a seven-level descriptor of reflective progression, which, although highly theoretical, is nonetheless useful.

Smith and Hatton (1993) describe three types of reflection, which move from descriptive to dialogic to critical. Conversely, Richardson (1995) introduces a way of seeing reflective development as multi-faceted and not linear or hierarchical. This has some face value, considering that it is clear that some students have a greater potential for reflective practice than others. It allows for a more individual and inclusive approach with multiple 'entry' and 'exit' points. Unfortunately, it is a difficult conceptual model to translate into assessment criteria. Nevertheless, one should try to assess students' starting points individually, and recognise that some progress more quickly and further than others.

Issues for students and teaching staff in the assessment of reflection

The difficulties that staff and students find in the assessment of reflection mirror the broader problems. A study by C.J. Angove (unpublished observations, 1999) explored the perspectives of academic staff in the assessment of reflection, and found that these people held equivocal views of what they were actually assessing. A major area of concern was the correlation between good reflective writing and its translation into practice; this is echoed by other authors (for example, Stewart and Richardson 2000). Also, some staff were not clear about how grading criteria related to levels of reflection and this influenced the guidance that students received. There are a number of issues here that may have a negative impact on the reliability of an assessment tool; and it is clear that agreed values, consistent support and feedback, and adequate preparation of staff assessing reflection are important. These issues are congruent with the findings of Stewart and Richardson (2000) who explored the experiences of occupational therapy and physiotherapy students. In this study, both staff and students had reservations about the assessment of reflection, and, again, levels of support for students varied. Following their findings, Stewart and Richardson proposed more of a focus on the *process* of reflection, rather than the outcome. This gives some support to the use of levels of reflection and to the use of self-assessment in order to move students through the levels.

King and Kitchener (1994) developed a model of reflective judgment from their work with college students. They suggested that students' ability to manage their college work depends partly on *the recognition that issues can be ill defined and demand reflective judgment*. In fact, we as nurses would recognise this in practice – we just need to translate the understanding into reflecting on the process of reflection. Of course, this echoes the original work of Schön (1983, 1987) who described these aspects of professional practice as the *swampy lowlands*. King and Kitchener's model has seven stages whereby assumptions about the

nature of knowledge increase in sophistication with accompanying development of the ability to reflect on poorly structured situations:

- Pre-reflective stages:
  - Stage one: knowledge is absolute.
  - Stage two: knowledge is absolute but not always immediately available.
  - Stage three: knowledge is absolute in the majority of cases, but briefly uncertain in others.

- Quasi-reflective stages:
  - Stage four: knowledge is uncertain, as there is always a constituent of ambiguity in evidence.
  - Stage five: knowledge is personal, since individuals must interpret the evidence.

- Reflective stages:
  - Stage six: knowledge concerning ill-structured problems is constructed by appraising other's evidence.
  - Stage seven: knowledge of ill-structured problems is constructed from inquiry, which leads to sensible solutions based on currently available evidence.

This model has some potential for dealing with negative experiences of staff and students in the assessment of reflection. King and Kitchener (1994) suggest that first-year students could be expected to be at level three to four, whilst senior students could be expected to be at level four. Thus a qualifying nurse may only reach the quasi-reflective stage at entry to primary practice. This may be a useful means of overcoming the fear that many experienced practitioners have of reflection, as so many cannot see their own inherent reflective abilities when they are asked to engage in reflection, or feel that they are engaging in reflection when they are not. In formal courses, linking this to grading criteria may be useful, but, more importantly, the model could be used to help both assessors and students to come to terms with the ambiguities and lack of definition in what is being assessed.

What assessors and teachers of reflection need to come to terms with is the fact that their role is of 'guide on the side' rather than 'sage on the stage' (Durgahee 1998). Thus teachers and assessors are facilitators rather than anything else. Facilitation is, supposedly, widely accepted in nurse education, yet it seems likely that this less than distinct role is actually what is causing the problems here. Teachers are often asked to be both facilitators and assessors of reflection and this can cause tensions at best and conflict at worst.

Evaluating reflection

As reflection becomes integrated within nurse education, it is increasingly important to demonstrate the benefits for professional practice and health and social care delivery. It is only through effective evaluation that this impact can be quantified. It is argued that all educational activity needs evaluation (Herbener and Watson 1992), and indeed, as students and educators, it is a large part of our daily lives. With the growing use of reflection in both pre- and post-registration programmes over the past decade, evaluation of this approach is well overdue. Whilst reflection is perceived to play a key role in the development of effective practitioners of nursing, there is a lack of empirical evidence to support the assertion that engaging in reflective practice actually changes or in any way benefits patient care (Andrews *et al.* 1998). This highlights the need for evaluation strategies that focus specifically on the link between educational programmes and clinical effectiveness (Jordan 1988). However, the situated, contextually bound benefits to practice that may result from reflective practice cannot often be labelled as 'clinically effective'.

Thus, evaluating reflection and reflective practice needs to be seen more in context. How can a nurse's development in practice, as an outcome of reflective activity, be measured? Whilst reflective assessments as part of an overall assessment strategy can be quantified using grading systems such as those described above, this alone is not sufficient. We need to address the pervasive anxiety about whether good reflective writing equals good reflective practice. Writing about practice development as a result of reflection may not equate with actual practice development as we have seen, let alone be a direct consequence of reflection. We must also recognise that measuring the practice development of an individual is fraught with difficulties, as so many other variables may have an influence. As Heath (1998) points out, reflection as a concept does not lend itself to the research approaches that can make such a measurement anyway.

As a first step, it is useful to consider the potential outcomes of reflection, as this will help to inform potential evaluation criteria. Boud *et al.* (1985) suggested that the outcomes of reflection are both cognitive and affective in nature, and provided a list of potential outcomes summarised into four key areas:

1. new perspectives on experience;
2. change in behaviour;
3. readiness for application;
4. commitment to action.

Reflective learning then may be evaluated by measuring the extent to which a student has a changed perspective on practice as a result of experience. This change in perspective may also lead to changes in attitudes, values and consequently, behaviour. The learner should demonstrate motivation to apply new knowledge and skills in practice. There may also be a deepening of understanding of the learner's own learning style and needs, with a positive attitude towards further learning. Reflection should be a journey that spirals into deeper reflection; see Sue Duke's discussion of her experience of this (Chapter 8) and you will see how measuring the outcomes of reflection may not be a straightforward activity. Boud et al. (1985) recognised that some of these outcomes are intangible and may not be easily demonstrated or observed in the practice completion of an educational programme. Thus, questions emerge about the most effective strategy for accurately measuring outcomes of reflection and therefore for evaluating its success.

Whilst the issue of evaluating reflective learning is recognised in the literature, a limited number of studies have been conducted in this area. Strategies that can be utilised include:

- qualitative evaluation by assessors and students;
- surveys collecting quantitative evaluation data;
- meta-analysis of data from student assessments of a reflective nature;
- qualitative and quantitative evaluation of student performance in a reflective practice setting where students are placed.

The main focus of this type of evaluation is to find the degree to which there is a change in a student's or practitioner's action as a demonstration of new knowledge or new skills. The key issue in terms of approach is to ask and also observe, so that what is espoused and what is actually present in practice are both evaluated.

Exploration is likely to be made around the following criteria:

1. development of the knowledge base;
2. development of new skills or the advancement of previous skills;
3. a change in or refining of attitudes and values;
4. participation in reflective activities;
5. clinical practice development initiatives.

This approach relies heavily on individual perceptions of development in practice and this may not be an effective method of evaluation due to inter-rater reliability issues. Utilising exemplars from practice to illustrate the measurement of criteria above can contribute towards the veracity of findings, much as the use of participants' own words does in qualitative research. Approaches such as Fourth Generation Evaluation (Guba and Lincoln 1989) may be a valuable way in which to consider evaluation of reflection. This strategy utilises the methodology of qualitative inquiry to collect and evaluate data from the perspectives of stakeholders (those

Chapter 3

experiencing the phenomenon). This would include patients, families, nursing staff, students, medical and allied health professionals, facilitators and mentors.

Andrews *et al.* (1998) asserted that patient outcomes should be included in evaluating reflective practice to determine if the benefits of reflection are transmitted to patient outcomes. Without this, the cycle is not complete, although this is likely to be some time coming. No clear evidence has yet been presented through good quality research that reflection by health and social care staff makes any difference to patient outcomes. Durgahee (1998) suggested that patients' perceptions of reflective practitioners should be included in the evaluation of reflective practice – that would be a truly interesting study. Research of this nature, although needed, demands some considerable skill by a researcher and there would need to be robust research strategies in place to achieve this. Yet Rome was not built in a day and less sophisticated areas need attention before we are ready to approach this one. The need to evaluate the benefits of reflection is closely allied to the need to evaluate how it is facilitated and assessed. There are some particular imperatives:

- the need to identify strategies that will map change in practice over time as a result of reflective practice as distinct from other variables;
- how to include patients' perspectives in the evaluation;
- the need for long-term studies that will elicit the effects of reflection on practitioners over time.

It is clearly very important that where reflection is assessed, the relative merits of assessment strategies and their levels of success are evaluated. In the earlier parts of this chapter, evaluation and assessment were defined as being two distinct activities, but it is clearly the case that where one is attempted, the other must be too. Evaluation of an assessment strategy must involve both placing a relative value on it and measuring its success.

Conclusion

In this chapter I have debated what is meant by the terms assessment and evaluation in relation to reflection. Definitions have been put forward and the contextual issues discussed. I have highlighted some of the philosophical issues that arise when attempting to assess reflection and have offered a perspective on these. The challenges associated with assessment of reflection have been indicated and some practical solutions suggested. Tools that are available for assessment are outlined, with a discussion of some of the relative benefits and issues. The evaluation of reflective practice is also discussed and some research priorities offered. In summary, reflective practice is a means to enhance effective interventions with patients and clients in nursing. Reflection is therefore central to nurse education and must be treated as such. This involves making clear and unambiguous assessment of the abilities of those engaged in reflection and working at developing these over time. Evaluating the efficacy of these strategies is vital in order to instigate change and progress the art and science of reflective practice.

Acknowledgements

I would like to thank Pam Sharp, Carrie Angove and Chris Bulman for their contributions to this chapter.

References

Andrews, M., Gidman, J. and Humphreys, A. (1998) Reflection: does it enhance professional nursing practice? *British Journal of Nursing*, **7** (7), 413–417.

Ashford, D., Blake, D., Knott, C., Platzer, H. and Snelling, J. (1998) Changing conceptions of reflective practice in social work, health and education. An institutional case study. *Journal of Interprofessional Care*, **12** (1), 7–19.

Bolton, G. (2005) *Reflective Writing*, 2nd edn. Paul Chapman, London.

Boud, D., Keogh, R. and Walker, D. (eds) (1985) *Reflection: Turning Experience into Learning*. Kogan Page, London.

Burnard, P. (1988) The journal as an assessment tool in nurse education. *Nurse Education Today*, **8**, 105–107.

Burnard, P. (1995) Nurse educators' perceptions of reflection and reflective practice: a report of the descriptive study. *Journal of Advanced Nursing*, **21**, 1167–1174.

Burns, S. (1994) Assessing reflective learning. In: *Reflective Practice in Nursing: The Growth of the Professional Practitioner* (eds A. Palmer, S. Burns and C. Bulman). Blackwell Scientific Publications, Oxford.

Burrows, D.E. (1995) The nurse teacher's role in the promotion of reflective practice. *Nurse Education Today*, **15**, 346–350.

Burton, A.J. (2000) Reflection: nursing's practice and education panacea? *Journal of Advanced Nursing*, **31** (5), 1009–1017.

Cotton, A.H. (2001) Private thoughts in the public sphere: issues in reflection and reflective practice in nursing. *Journal of Advanced Nursing*, **36** (4), 512–519.

Daly, W. (1998) Critical thinking as an outcome of nursing education. What is it? Why is it important to nursing practice? *Journal of Advanced Nursing*, **28**, 323–331.

Durgahee, T. (1998) Facilitating reflection: from a sage on a stage to a guide on the side. *Nurse Education Today*, **18**, 158–164.

Eraut, M. (1994) *Developing Professional Knowledge and Competence*. Routledge Falmer, London.

Flannigan, J.C. (1954) The critical incident technique. *Psychological Bulletin*, **51**, 327–358.

Fund, Z., Court, D. and Kramarski, B. (2002) Construction and application of an evaluative tool to assess reflection in teacher-training courses. *Assessment and Evaluation in Higher Education*, **27** (6), 481–499.

Getliffe, K.A. (1996) An examination of the use of reflection in the assessment of practice for undergraduate nursing students. *International Journal of Nursing Studies*, **33** (4), 361–374.

Ghaye, Y. and Lillyman, S. (2000) *Reflection: Principles and Practice for Health Care Professionals*. Mark Allen Publishing, London.

Gibbs, G., Farmer, B. and Eastcott, D. (1988) *Learning by Doing. A Guide to Teaching and Learning Methods*, pp.46–47. FEU, Birmingham Polytechnic.

Glaze, J.E. (2002) Stages in coming to terms with reflection: student advanced nurse practitioners' perceptions of their reflective journeys. *Journal of Advanced Nursing*, **37** (30), 265–272.

Goodman, J. (1984) Reflection and teacher education: a case study and theoretical analysis. *Interchange*, **15** (3), 9–26.

Greenwood, J. (1998) The role of reflection in single and double loop learning. *Journal of Advanced Nursing*, **27** (5), 1048–1053.

Guba, E.G. and Lincoln, D.Y.S. (1989) *Fourth Generation Evaluation*. Sage, Thousand Oaks.

Hannigan, B. (2001) A discussion of the strengths and weaknesses of 'reflection' in nursing practice and education. *Journal of Clinical Nursing*, **10**, 278–283.

Heath, H. (1998) Reflection and patterns of knowing in nursing. *Journal of Advanced Nursing*, **27**, 1054–1059.

Herbener, D. and Watson, J. (1992) Models for evaluating nurse education programmes. *Nursing Outlook*, **40** (1), 27–32.

James, C.R. and Clarke, B.A. (1994) Reflective practice in nursing: issues for nurse education. *Nurse Education Today*, **14**, 82–90.

Johns, C. (1995) The value of reflective practice for nursing. *Journal of Clinical Nursing*, **4**, 23–30.

Johns, C. (2005) *Guided Reflection*. Blackwell Science, Oxford.

Johns, C. and Freshwater, D. (1998) *Transforming Nursing Through Reflective Practice*. Blackwell Science, Oxford.

Jordan, S. (1988) From classroom theory to clinical practice: evaluating the impact of a post-registration course. *Nurse Education Today*, **18**, 293–302.

Kember, D., Jones, A., Loke, A.Y., *et al.* (2001) Encouraging reflective writing. In: *Reflective Teaching and Learning in the Health Professions* (eds D. Kember *et al.*). Blackwell Science, Oxford.

King, P.M. and Kitchener, K.S. (1994) *Developing Reflective Judgement: Understanding and Promoting Intellectual Growth and Critical Thinking in Adolescents and Adults*. Jossey Bass, San Francisco.

Korthagen, F.A.J. and Wubbels, T. (1995) Characteristics of reflective practitioners: towards an operationalisation of the concept of reflection. *Teachers and Teaching: Theory and Practice*, **1** (1), 51–72.

Lowe, P.B. and Kerr, C.M. (1998) Learning by reflection: the effect on educational outcomes. *Journal of Advanced Nursing*, **27**, 1030–1033.

Mackintosh, C. (1998) Reflection: a flawed strategy for the nursing profession. *Nurse Education Today*, **18**, 553–557.

Mallik, M. (1998) The role of nurse educators in the development of reflective practitioners: a selective case study of the Australian and UK experience. *Nurse Education Today*, **18** (1), 52–63.

Mezirow, J. (1991) *Transformative Dimensions of Adult Learning*. Jossey Bass, San Francisco.

Morgan, R. and Johns, C. (2005) The beast and the star: resolving contradictions in everyday practice: In: *Transforming Nursing Through Reflective Practice* (ed. C. Johns), 2nd edn, Chapter 9. Blackwell Publishing, Oxford.

Mountford, B. and Rogers, L. (1996) Using individual and group reflection in and on assessment as a tool for effective learning. *Journal of Advanced Nursing*, **24**, 1127–1134.

Newell, R. (1994) Reflection: art, science or pseudo-science? (Editorial). *Nurse Education Today*, **14**, 79–81.

Norman, I., Redfern, S., Tomalin, D., and Oliver, S. (1992) Developing Flannigan's critical incident technique to elicit indicators of high and low quality nursing care from patients and their nurses. *Journal of Advanced Nursing*, **17**, 590–600.

Paget, T. (2001) Reflective practice and clinical outcomes: practitioners' views on how reflective practice has influenced their clinical practice. *Journal of Clinical Nursing*, **10**, 204–214.

Perry, L. (1997) Critical incidents, crucial issues: insights into the working lives of registered nurses. *Journal of Clinical Nursing*, **6**, 131–137.

Phillips, T., Schostak, J. and Tyler, J. (2000) *Practice and Assessment in Nursing and Midwifery: Doing it for Real*. English National Board for Nursing, Midwifery and Health Visiting, Researching Professional Education Series, London.

Platzer, H., Blake, D. and Ashford, D. (2000) Barriers to learning from reflection: a study of the use of group-work with post-registration nurses. *Journal of Advanced Nursing*, **31** (5), 1001–1008.

Powell, J. (1989) The reflective practitioner in nursing. *Journal of Advanced Nursing*, **14**, 824–832.

Reece-Jones, P. (1995) Hindsight bias in reflective practice: an empirical investigation. *Journal of Advanced Nursing*, **21** (4), 783–788.

Rich, A. and Parker, D. (1995) Reflection and critical incident analysis: ethical and moral implications of their use within nursing and midwifery education. *Journal of Advanced Nursing*, **22**, 1050–1057.

Richardson, G. and Maltby, H. (1995) Reflection on practice: enhancing student learning. *Journal of Advanced Nursing*, **22**, 235–242.

Richardson, R. (1995) Humpty Dumpty: reflection and reflective nursing practice. *Journal of Advanced Nursing*, **21**, 1044–1050.

Rolfe, G., Freshwater, D. and Jasper, M. (2001) *Critical Reflection for Nursing and the Helping Professions*. Palgrave, Basingstoke.

Schön, D. (1983) *The Reflective Practitioner*. Jossey Bass, San Francisco.

Schön, D.A. (1987) *Educating the Reflective Practitioner*. Jossey Bass, San Francisco.

Schutz, S., Bulman, C. and Salussolia, M. (1996) The learning contract as a tool for documenting competence. *Teaching News* (Oxford Brookes University), **43**, 17–18.

Smith, D. and Hatton, N. (1993) Reflection in teacher education: a study in progress. *Education Research and Perspectives*, **20** (1), 13–23.

Smith, A. and Russell, J. (1991) Using critical incidents in nurse education. *Nurse Education Today*, **11** (4), 284–291.

Stewart, S. and Richardson, B. (2000) Reflection and its place in the curriculum: should it be assessed? *Assessment and Evaluation in Higher Education*, **25** (4), 369–380.

Sumison, J. and Fleet, A. (1996) Reflection: can we assess it? *Assessment and Evaluation in Higher Education*, **21** (2), 121–130.

Wallace, D. (1996) Experiential learning and critical thinking in nursing. *Nursing Standard*, **10** (31), 43–47.

Wittgenstein, L. (1967) *Philosophical Investigations*. Blackwell, Oxford.

Wong, F., Kember, D., Chung, L. and Yan, L. (1995) Assessing the level of student reflection from reflective journals. *Journal of Advanced Nursing*, **22**, 48–57.

Zeichner, K.M. and Liston, D.P. (1987) Teaching student teachers to reflect. *Harvard Educational Review*, **57** (1), 23–48.

Chapter 4

An exploration of the student and mentor journey into reflective practice

Pam Sharp and Charlotte Maddison

Introduction

Health and social care is in a state of constant change and nursing is not immune to the impact of these changes. The Royal College of Nursing (RCN 2004) outlined some of the ongoing issues, including: an aging population, changes to services, public expectations, advances in technology and a need to increase the efficiency and effectiveness of health and social care. They identified that the supply of an appropriately trained workforce is key to this, as is the need to balance the demand for nursing care with the predicted supply of nurses. Hall (2006) commented that the workforce shortages provide an opportunity to reflect on how to further develop placements. Wagner (2007) (President of the International Council of Nurses), at an international conference on nurse education, highlighted how the global shortage of nurses had significant implications for education. Nurses need to be aware of such influences on practice (Taylor 2006), that the nursing workforce has changed and that there is a current shortage of recruits, with all the impact that this brings (Edmond 2001). This inevitably places pressures on practice education as there are fewer mentors/supervisors available in practice and those that are available are under greater time constraints (Magnusson et al. 2007; Mallik and McGowan 2007). Some of these changes have impacted on placement learning, as both the Quality Assurance Agency (QAA) (2001) and Chapple and Aston (2004) note. The Nursing and Midwifery Council (NMC 2006) has acknowledged that Higher Education Institutions (HEIs) need to work in partnership with placement providers to ensure that learning outcomes can be achieved.

Burton (2000), in an article entitled 'Reflection: nursing's practice and education panacea?', concluded that despite criticism, reflection has a place in educational programmes, because there is no real alternative way to help nurses think critically before, during and after practice. On a more positive note, Turner and Beddoes (2007) asserted that reflection is the cornerstone of nursing practice. From our own personal experiences we are convinced that introducing, developing and using reflection within the university setting and within placements helps both students and practitioners on their professional journey towards excellent practice and life-long learning.

This chapter outlines the student's journey into reflection, including how the skills for reflection are acquired as part of the student's academic skills development and to prepare him or her for practice placement. The mentor's journey in supporting, facilitating and assessing student learning using reflection will be examined and the potential for 'reflective opportunities' in practice will be explored. Consequently this chapter adds to the work on skills for reflection and on the assessment of reflection given in other chapters of this book. Throughout this chapter we provide examples taken predominantly from work with pre-registration students and their mentors, although some of the areas of discussion equate equally to those in post-qualifying education. Additionally, more experienced practitioners may wish to read Chapter 5 by Jane M. Appleton, who further explores reflection in post-qualifying education.

The NMC (2006) Standards to Support Learning and Assessment in Practice have been produced following wide consultation on the standards themselves and on *fitness to practice* at the point of registration (UKCC 1999; NMC 2005). The NMC sees its role as 'protecting the public' and the production of standards as a way of fulfilling this aim. The key aim for placement learning is to develop students who are 'fit for practice' (UKCC 1999) and to furnish learners with skills for life-long learning. The UK Department of Health (DH) (2001) noted the need for nurses to be equipped to work in a rapidly changing context and therefore life-long learning has never been so important. In the UK, the Department of Health (DH 2004) National Health Service Knowledge and Skills Framework (NHS KSF), which contributes to formulating an outline for each post in the NHS, describes how the 'development review' process is an ongoing cycle of learning that consists of evaluating learning and development and reflecting on how it has been applied. Gould et al. (2007) gave a clear overview of the implications and importance of the NHS KSF for clinicians and educational providers. A portfolio of evidence including reflection-on-practice forms part of this process. Reflection is identified specifically in core dimension 2: 'Personal and People Development', where it is described as being part of 'on-the-job' learning through professional or clinical supervision and personal reflection. Reflection is also identified as part of developing communication skills and quality and service development. Jasper (2006, p.48) outlined a professional development triangle that indicates the place of reflection in this process (Fig. 4.1).

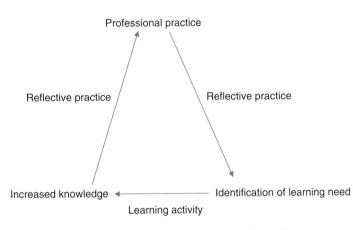

Fig. 4.1   Professional development triangle (Jasper 2006, p.48)

Hargreaves (2004) pointed out that the concept of reflection has been widely accepted as a valid and essential part of professional development. The NMC (2004, p.34) Standards of Proficiency for Pre-Registration Nursing Education which outline the competencies required for registration include (under the domain of personal and professional development) the need for students who enter onto the register to:

'. . . identify one's own professional development needs by engaging in activities such as reflection in and on practice and life long learning'.

Readers may like to look at the NMC website (www.nmc.org) to find the results of the consultation on the future of pre-registration nurse education, undertaken during December 2007 to February 2008.

Clouder and Sellers (2004) and Racey (2005) noted that it is clear that supervision and reflection are inextricably linked. The NMC Code of Conduct is being updated at time of going to press; however, the current version says that nurses must:

'. . . facilitate students and others to develop their competence' and '. . . must take part in appropriate learning and practice activities that maintain and develop (your) competence and performance'. (NMC 2007a, p.3)

Therefore qualified staff will have responsibility for engaging in learning activities for the benefit of students and for their own personal and professional development.

The student's journey into reflection

Many pre-registration students will enter higher education with little or no exposure to reflection as a concept. When asked, they state that 'it is just something you do', reinforcing Reid's (1993) observation in the title of her paper 'But we're doing it already!' When students enter what can be a diverse and complex range of clinical placements they will inevitably experience a variety of situations that evoke a range of emotional responses, necessitating them to be equipped with ways of learning from these experiences. Even if a student has had prior exposure to, or experience of, working within health and social care, it cannot be assumed that the student will find it easy to gain the knowledge and skills necessary to practice safely and competently. However, needs may vary. In order for learning to take place both in the university and practice setting, a student needs purposeful structure to the learning experiences, which must include reflection upon that experience (Brackenbreg 2004). This would mean integrating the development of such skills as critical thinking, self-awareness, problem-solving and analysis into the curriculum, as outlined in Chapter 2.

By having the opportunity to reflect upon a particular learning activity or experience the student can more easily make links between theory and practice (O'Regan and Fawcett 2006). Jasper (2006) noted that reflection can be used as a strategy that involves thinking about practice experiences, in order to help develop understanding and so inform practice. She outlined three stages of reflective practice: experience, reflection and action. The ultimate aim in helping students to reflect is therefore to influence their actual performance as practitioners.

Preparation for nursing practice in pre-registration programmes occurs through a variety of means and students will learn about nursing by engaging in different learning activities. These may involve role-play, discussion around case studies, simulated activities in the skills laboratory and experience in practice. Both Jasper (2006) and Fowler (2007) undertook an exploration of the literature and discussed the concept of experience-based learning. They acknowledged previous work (Kolb 1984) and suggested that learning will only take place if an experience and an opportunity to reflect are both present. Irrespective of the delivery method, students will achieve the greatest learning if they are able to reflect upon the educational activity. We think this is particularly relevant to practice-related learning and to those that supervise it. To enable students to reflect, Brackenbreg (2004) has discussed the importance of teaching staff being able to facilitate effectively.

It is evident that students benefit from being able to reflect upon experiences (Green 2002; Pfund et al. 2003; Bulman 2004; O'Donovan 2005; O'Regan and Fawcett 2006). However, students will require preparation if they are to utilise the skill successfully (O'Donovan 2005).

Preparation should include establishing the purpose and benefits of reflection and its relevance to the students in both the practice setting and their academic work and in fact to their lives in general. In the previous edition of this book, Maddison (2004) made reference to Knowles's (1990) theory of adult learning, which asserts that learners need to know *why* knowledge is necessary in order to accept it. This is no different for reflective practice. Relevance may be achieved by making connections with how and where students will use reflection in the educational programmes, in practice and in their personal development.

There are many ways of introducing reflection to students through interactive, self-directed, blended or taught approaches to learning. Students are presented with a variety of reflective frameworks and are encouraged to identify one that suits them. This is often a daunting proposition for students given the increasing number of reflective frameworks available. Often students will opt for Gibbs *et al.* (1988) as it is seen to provide a relatively simple and logical process through reflection. However, an exploration of alternative frameworks should be encouraged as students become more experienced in reflection. The final chapter of this book also gives advice and further reading on the use of these frameworks.

Within our pre-registration programmes, group tutorials, facilitated by the students' personal tutors, take place throughout the academic year. These offer an opportunity for students to develop the skills required for reflection, which are self-awareness, description, critical analysis, synthesis and evaluation, as described in Chapter 2. The approaches we use for the development of these skills will now be examined further.

Developing self-awareness

It would be wrong to expect student nurses to become self-aware merely by presenting them with the theory. A good place to start is by asking students to carry out a self-assessment that relates to a particular skill or action. Self-assessment requires self-awareness and is regarded as a lifelong skill. Professional practitioners have a responsibility to assess their own competence. Price (2005) and Levett-Jones and Bourgeois (2007) argued that students should be given the opportunity to self-assess their clinical ability and competence throughout their programme. As part of the pre-registration programme at our university, students are asked to self-assess in a variety of ways. Initially they focus on transferable skills: qualities and attributes acquired during previous life experience. Examples of such transferable skills are teamwork, communication, information technology skills and time management.

When in practice, students are asked to carry out self-assessment of their achievement of the specific clinical competencies required for the placement. This self-assessment can form the basis of discussions between the mentor and the student regarding the student's progress in achieving specific clinical competencies. This will be discussed in greater depth later. This self-assessment will form part of the student's portfolio of evidence, or what the NMC (2006, p.30) refers to as the 'student passport'.

Self-awareness is imperative for effective practice learning and development and has to be developed whilst actually in practice. However, as a result of concerns raised about the level of competence of newly registered nurses (UKCC 1999), an ever more overburdened workforce and scarcity of placements (Hall 2006), clinical skills teaching in the 'simulated clinical environment' is becoming increasingly common (Chatterjee 2004; Hilton and Pollard 2004; Wilson *et al.* 2005). At Oxford Brookes University, the teaching of clinical skills is fundamental to all practice modules and students are introduced to an ever-increasing range of clinical activities. This is a focus emphasised in the NMC (2007b) skills clusters. In the simulated clinical setting students are able to practice clinical and professional skills in a safe environment where awareness of their own limitations and strengths can be developed under supervision. Prior to attending a session, they are asked to carry out a self-assessment of the skill. For some programmes this is a requirement or part of the assessment process. The form below is used by students before and after each skills session in order to promote reflection.

Clinical skills: self-assessment form
Before the activity

- What knowledge do I have of the topic area?
- Where has the knowledge come from?
- What practical experience do I have of this topic area?
- Was I aware of the theory and the relevant standards when I practiced this in the past?
- What are my hopes in completing these workstations?

After the activity:

- What new knowledge have I gained?
- Did I work well with my group and support and share with them?
- How well did I practice my skills?
- What could I have done better?
- What is my plan of action for my future practice with regard to this topic?

The questions above can act as triggers that enable the student to identify knowledge, thoughts and assumptions that may guide future learning. Self-assessment alone does not guarantee self-awareness; therefore students are reminded of the value in checking whether their self-assessment matches the view of others and of asking for specific feedback.

In order to further help students develop their self-awareness, we utilise various exercises and activities. Some of the activities are based upon the work of Rungapadiachy (1999) who suggested that there are three dimensions to self-awareness. The three dimensions are: cognitive (know yourself), affective (feel yourself) and behavioural (be yourself). These dimensions are not independent and will inevitably influence each other. Having an awareness of these concepts will help students to acknowledge and understand how their beliefs, feelings and actions might influence their response to an experience or situation.

In tutor groups, we draw upon Rungapadiachy's (1999, p.18) dimensions described above and ask students to identify a situation and consider whether their:

1. **behaviour** has influenced their **thoughts**
2. **thought** has influenced their **behaviour**
3. **behaviour** has influenced their **feeling**

Example: self-awareness

When carrying out this activity, one student described the action of answering the telephone whilst in her placement. She described how she answered the ward telephone (**behaviour**). The person making the call was a member of staff from another department who (according to the student) was surprised that a student had answered the call and asked to speak to a qualified member of staff. Based upon this she assumed (**thought**) that students should not answer the telephone. Consequently based on that experience she would not answer the telephone in her clinical placements. The student stated that she was not confident (**feeling**) to answer the ward telephone. This exercise enabled the student to acknowledge how her previous behaviour and thoughts had influenced her feeling about that particular activity and that this had resulted in problems in subsequent placements.

Carrying out this self-awareness exercise enabled the student to begin the process of reflection and she could go on to further analyse her own assumptions and actions.

How do students know if they are self-aware?

We all think we have a good awareness of self. However, the only way we can truly know this is to actively seek out specific and honest feedback. The Johari window (Luft and Ingham 1955, cited in Rungapadiachy 1999; Fig. 4.2) may help students to become more aware of themselves

1. Open area	2. Blind area
What is known by the person about him/herself and is also known by others – open area, open self, free area, free self or 'the arena'	What is unknown by the person about him/herself but which others know – blind area, blind self or 'blind spot'
3. Hidden area	4. Unknown area
What the person knows about him/herself that others do not know – hidden area, hidden self, avoided area, avoided self or 'facade'	What is unknown by the person about him/herself and is also unknown by others – unknown area or unknown self

Fig. 4.2   Johari window (adapted from Luft and Ingham 1955)

and to understand particularly how they may function within a group by considering the four areas in the window:

- Area 1: can be seen as the space where good communication and cooperation occur without conflict and misunderstanding.
- Area 2: can be developed by seeking feedback from others in order to reduce the blind area and thereby increase the open area.
- Area 3: where certain information and feelings should remain hidden which have no bearing on work. However, typically some information is work or performance-related, and so is better positioned in the open area. Development of trust between individuals and establishing boundaries or ground-rules can help individuals feel safer in disclosing these hidden areas.
- Area 4: the uncovering of this area is personal and not always appropriate as part of a learning activity. However, this emerging knowledge of self can be uncovered through deeper analysis and sometimes counselling.

In order to enhance students' self-awareness of their clinical skills, audio-visual recording is used to help students to review and reflect upon their practice. When practicing hand-washing techniques, the students are filmed (with their consent). Following the activity, students are asked to reflect on and self-assess their performance. Often students are unaware if they have omitted a stage of the hand-washing procedure. The footage is then played back to the students, which challenges their perception and helps them to realise areas that require more practice. As a result it brings areas for development to the surface.

Sully and Dallas (2005) say that self-awareness in communication can help us to develop empathy, recognise our perceptions of our clients and cope with distractions, enabling us to develop further the attentive listening skills we need. In order to promote this with our students, we undertake the following activity:

Example: self-awareness activity

When learning communication skills, students are asked to practice active listening. This involves being in a triad. One student is given a topic to discuss (i.e. his or her first week at university), another is asked to demonstrate active listening and the third student acts as an observer, giving feedback on the listener's performance. Students who found this useful did so because they realised that their own perception was different from the observer. For example, a student might have thought that 'I looked interested and focused' whereas the observer may comment that 'You fiddled with your pen and occasionally your eyes seemed to glaze over'.

We often need the perspective of another to challenge our self-awareness and Brookfield (2001) has discussed the need to consider different perspectives when exploring our own beliefs and assumptions. However, it is often difficult to step outside our own point of view. In the exercise above, the observer can reflect the actions back to the students, giving them the opportunity to view what they did from a different perspective. The observer is, in essence, acting as a mirror to the students (Brookfield 2001).

Mirroring of students' behaviour or assumptions will take place in a variety of situations. Some pre-registration students (for example those students studying in the mental health or midwifery fields) will experience clinical supervision (Clouder and Sellers 2004), bringing with it an opportunity to reflect on practice with a peer and so gain an alternative perspective. Challenge of one's own perspective by another is key here (Daloz 1986) and a skilled facilitator or mentor will stretch students to consider how they self-assessed or evaluated their own performance and more importantly how they 'checked out' their assumptions.

Developing descriptive skills

When exploring the purpose and reasons for reflection with students, they seem to recognise that it can help them to review an incident and learn from practice experiences (Jasper 2006). However, students tend to focus on feelings and often just write descriptively. The idea of describing concisely as well as identifying the important issues may be a challenge for some. Often the focus is on helping students to develop their descriptive skills in the written form, for example, through the use of diaries, as described by Melanie Jasper in Chapter 7, through portfolios (McMullan 2006) or in academic essays. A concern expressed by Platzer *et al.* (1997), particularly in relation to journal writing, is that practitioners

Chapter 4

may never move from the descriptive stage of reflection. Harris (2007) acknowledged the difficulties that students may face when writing and suggested that structured support is necessary to help students learn from their reflective writing. It can take time for students to benefit from their writing and there is a risk that they will opt out of reflection if it becomes seen as a largely academic activity. Helping students to describe well in writing may equip them to articulate verbally and vice versa, and so individual learning styles or preferences (Kolb and Fry 1975; Honey and Mumford 2000; Fleming 2007) should be considered.

Levett-Jones (2007, p.112) defined a narrative approach as 'a brief account of an actual situation or episode in practice that is significant because it resulted in new learning and or new understanding'. She outlined the benefits of a narrative approach as being:

- learn from practice through reflection;
- describe and critically analyse episodes of clinical practice;
- illuminate and assess own level of competence;
- identify areas of strength and those requiring development;
- develop practice-driven learning objectives.

In situations where a student's description is superficial, the teacher or mentor can help him or her to develop these skills by providing a balance of challenge and support (Daloz 1986). Asking students how they validated or 'checked out' their assumptions can challenge the accuracy of the description, which can become more concise if students are asked for the relevance of the content. Support is important here to ensure that students do not feel anxious about what they are being asked to describe, which could result in the student withdrawing from the activity. A verbal narrative can be developed in practice and in the classroom through the mentor or teacher asking the student to describe events or incidents. Students can be encouraged by a facilitator asking them to '**tell me about it**' or '**tell me more about it**'. This can help develop students' verbal description skills.

Example: bed making

In a seminar group, students were reflecting in small groups about their recent practice experiences. One student commented that 'I didn't learn much yesterday, I seemed to be just making a lot of beds'. The facilitator asked her to '*tell me about it*'. Her detailed description was as follows:

'I was working with a care assistant and so we gathered the equipment that we needed. We washed our hands and put on

Contd.

aprons. We helped a patient out of bed (*the facilitator then asked her to elaborate more*). We assessed the patient's mobility and realised that with supervision they could move themselves and the positioning of the chair was important. I remembered the skills we had learnt in our manual handling session and so did not rush the patient but supported them to move themselves. We also talked to the patient about how they were feeling generally since their surgery, assessing pain and mobility in general. I think the patient appreciated the chat as she touched my arm as I helped her. Then we made the bed (*again the facilitator said 'tell me more about it'*). We put the bed up to a good height for both of us, we stripped the sheets off carefully to ensure minimal spreading of skin cells and bugs, we had brought the white linen skip to the bedside and put the soiled linen in it . . . I remember the fun we had in the skills laboratory sorting rubbish and linen into the correct containers, although I must remember to check out the local policy. I also remember the need to ensure the smoothness of sheets as wrinkles can contribute to skin problems. . . .'

This example shows that the student had demonstrated several examples of applying theory to practice and personal learning, including issues concerning patient assessment, standard precautions, therapeutic communication, prevention of pressure sores and manual handling. The facilitator went on to help the student further evaluate her learning and identify future learning needs and articulate how she could use this learning as evidence for achievement of competencies. This challenge and development of verbal description can then help the student identify what to write in her reflection on practice.

Developing critical analysis and evaluation

Critical analysis invokes fear in many students and is considered hard to grasp. This may be because the word 'critical' suggests that the intention is to find fault or to disapprove. However, analysis of a practice experience should be promoted as a positive activity that involves the breaking down of the event into manageable components in order that it can be more easily examined. Cottrell (2005) also noted that good critical thinkers often have well-developed self-awareness and so developing this early is crucial. Techniques for critical analysis need to be developed as part of a broader range of academic skills, and Cottrell (2005) has offered some useful and practical ways in which students can develop this way of thinking so that they may apply it to their writing. When critically analysing practice, a judgement on the specific event will be made. Often we ask students what was good and bad about the experience. Gibbs *et al.* (1988) expand on analysis in their reflective cycle, adding the question: 'What sense can you make of the situation?' Atkins and Schutz in Chapter 2 of this book also suggest that critical analysis should involve identifying existing knowledge, exploration of feelings, challenging of assumptions and the exploration of alternative approaches. Students are helped to develop this skill through academic writing activities, which are then marked using specific grading criteria outlining the requirements. Detailed and focused feedback is essential in order that students may develop these skills as they progress academically. For more discussion about assessing reflection, read Chapter 3 on assessment and evaluation.

It is often helpful for a student to talk through an event, as in critical incident analysis (Ghaye and Lillyman 1997; McGrath and Higgins 2006) or debriefing. The teacher can adopt the use of 'Socratic questioning' (Elder and Paul 1998, cited in Harris 2007), which is an approach designed to uncover the realities of a problem through a systematic process. When a teacher adopts this principle of questioning, he/she aims to check a student's viewpoint or thinking about a given subject. In this way, such an approach can help to uncover beliefs and assumptions. It can also enable the teacher to check the student's knowledge of a subject and develop critical thinking with the student. Harris (2007) adopted the principle to support students' learning through written journals.

McLoughlin and Darvill (2007) outlined the use of reflection in problem-based learning (PBL), which is an increasingly popular approach to student learning. Within PBL students reflect on the knowledge gained, problem resolution and the effectiveness of the group process. PBL aims to help students to reflect upon the process of learning as well as the outcome. It is interesting to note that Barrows (1986) referred to the messy practice situations used in PBL and how for health care practitioners this connects with real life situations. This clearly links with Schön's (1983) initial observations about the swampy lowlands of practice. Williams (2001) concluded from a review of the literature that practitioners exposed to PBL develop the ability to be reflective in their learning and this skill is developed through a facilitative approach. McCloughlin and Darvill (2007) have also outlined how PBL places practice at the centre of knowledge and learning and how reflection is a clear part of the process. It is clear that PBL uses critical analysis and evaluation and those adopting this approach may further develop these skills.

Having examined how the student is introduced to both the concept of reflection and the skills required we will now explore this from the mentor's perspective.

The mentor's journey into reflection

Nursing and midwifery students are required to undertake 50% of their programme in practice and the role of the mentor as an individual who 'facilitates, supervises and assesses students in the practice setting' (NMC 2006, p.44) is crucial to this process. The mentor's role includes a wide range of activities, as outlined by the NMC (2006, p.17):

- Organising and coordinating student learning activities in practice;
- Supervising students in learning situations and providing them with constructive feedback on their achievements;
- Setting and monitoring achievement of realistic learning objectives;
- Assessing total performance including skills, attitudes and behaviours;
- Providing evidence as required by programme providers of student achievement or lack of achievement;
- Liaising with others to provide feedback, identify any concerns about the students' performance and agree action as appropriate;
- Providing evidence for or acting as sign-off mentors with regard to making decisions about achievement of proficiency at the end of a programme.

All this outlines what is a complex and challenging role for staff whose key responsibility is for patient/client care. In order to facilitate mentors in understanding their responsibilities, the NMC (2006, p.49) has identified as part of its standards a developmental framework moving from registrant to mentor, practice teacher and then teacher. The NMC identifies eight domains for each of these roles:

1. Establishing effective working relationships
2. Facilitation of learning
3. Assessment and accountability
4. Evaluation of learning
5. Creating an environment for learning
6. Context of practice
7. Evidence-based practice
8. Leadership.

The standards document is challenging in its organisation and presentation. In order to apply the standards, some interpretation is needed. However, there is potentially considerable overlap of the domains. Under 'Facilitation of learning' it is stated that mentors need to:

✳ 'support students in critically reflecting upon their learning experiences in order to enhance future learning' (NMC 2006, p.18)

Although this a broad remit, it can be interpreted across other domains. Yet for mentors it is the only place that reflection is mentioned explicitly in the standards and it is disappointing that the value of reflection is not outlined elsewhere. Drawing on all of the eight domains, opportunities for reflection on placement will be explored further to highlight this.

Mentor preparation courses need to be validated by the NMC (2006), which also states that registrants who make judgements about whether a student has achieved the required standards of proficiency for safe and effective practice must have been prepared for their role to support and assess learning, and have met NMC-defined outcomes. In reality, these programmes vary considerably in content, method and length (Andrews and Wallis 1999; Mallik and McGowan 2007). Watson (2004) also outlined that there is sometimes confusion regarding the purpose of mentor preparation courses. Mallik and McGowan (2007), in a scoping exercise, compared the nature of practice education in five professions: dietetics, nursing, occupational therapy, physiotherapy and radiography (available at www.practicebasedlearning.org). They identified areas of good practice and common features of mentor preparation, but recognised that there were major inconsistencies in content, level, length, mode of delivery and audit. In a table outlining the most frequently agreed content for preparation programmes, areas such as roles and responsibilities, facilitation of learning and reflective practice (which was the joint fifth most frequently agreed area) were identified. In our own multi-professional mentor preparation programme at Oxford, the learning outcomes include:

- identify values, attitudes and influences relating to relationships and support of learners and demonstrate an anti-discriminatory approach;
- self-assess and seek feedback regarding own skills in order to develop personally and professionally;
- reflect on own experience in order to inform future practice.

All of these require a mentor to be self-aware, to self-assess and to adopt reflective approaches. On the mentor preparation programme, the summative assignment is to write a reflective essay entitled:

> 'Critical reflection on my learning about facilitating and assessing workplace/placement learning: including reflection on the session plan/observed session and learning from the module overall'.

The aim of the assignment is to help mentors become familiar with, or develop further, their own reflective skills. We provide an example of reflective writing (see below) and use it in the taught sessions to relate to the reflective frameworks and to discuss the skills for reflection.

Chapter 4

Example: a mentor's reflective writing for the assessment

Throughout this essay I will reflect on the learning I have had whilst undertaking the module. Reid (1993, p.305) defines reflection as 'a process of examining an experience of practice in order to give account, analyse, evaluate, and so inform learning about practice'. Although this is now quite a dated definition, I find it useful as it is explicit and focuses on learning in practice which for me, as a facilitator of learning, is highly relevant. Therefore, throughout this essay I will try to examine my own experiences of being a facilitator of learning and analyse if and how what I have learnt on the module has influenced my practice. I was very nervous before starting this course as I have not studied for 10 years and it was interesting in the first session where we discussed Adult Learning Theory (Knowles 1990) to recognise my own expectations. I was hoping we would be given lots of information and the teacher would explain exactly what I needed to do. I soon discovered that I needed to think more like an adult learner and be responsible for my own learning and use my experience. During our first session our facilitator highlighted that she had not actually taught us much, but had used our own experiences. Banning (2004) supports what Knowles says and explains that student learning needs can be met when teaching is facilitative rather than didactic and when the teacher recognised the learning needs, past experience, relevant application and individual styles of learning of students when designing activities. I now try to assess my students' learning before they start so I can draw on their previous experiences. I have done this by meeting with them and asking them about what they have done, how they best learn, previous placements, etc. In the past, I may have been a bit too keen to show the student what I know and may have even tried to teach them things they already know. Understanding learning styles is important too, as I discovered when a student I had in placement didn't seem to be learning skills very quickly. When we discussed it, it was because although he liked to learn with demonstration and practice such as in a kinaesthetic approach described by Fleming (2007) in the VARK learning preferences, he generally liked to read up on things first and found it tricky to do things he didn't fully understand and so his learning preference was read/write. This can also be related to Maslow's Hierarchy of Needs (Maslow 1987) as before he could learn he needed to feel safe and, for him, preparing in advance of practising the skill was part of this aspect. Now when I first meet the student I think about how I can further apply this new learning to my practice, for example. . . .

Mentors can select a reflective framework of their choice and guided reflection (Johns 2002) is used in each taught session so that they get used to verbalising their own learning.

As a facilitator of this course, one of us recalls that:

> 'I have shared personal reflection on my own learning and performance, so role-modelling what mentors themselves are being asked to do. The elusive skills of analysis, evaluation and synthesis are also role modelled in the classroom (for example, when referring to educational theory or definitions they will be 'pulled apart', compared and their sources critiqued). I may end a session by reflecting on what I think went well; what I may change for next time'.

The idea behind this is that the participants will see how verbalising learning and reflecting on one's own performance can help others to learn. It is intended that they will see the value of role modelling and do this in their own practice with their learners. In order to further explore the practical application of reflection in a practice situation, the next section explores how reflection can be used in practice.

Using reflective opportunities in practice

This section gives an overview of when and how a mentor and student can reflect on placement. The eight domains of the NMC (2006) standards will be broadly used to discuss how reflection is integral to placement learning.

Establishing effective relationships and creating an environment for learning

Development of effective relationships is an important area in practice education. Moore and Way (2004) in a report commissioned by the NMC summarised the three most important factors influencing students' experiences in placement:

1. the climate (welcoming, enquiring and reflective culture);
2. structure (clarity of learning opportunities);
3. attention (interested and skilled mentor).

To apply this to practice, mentors should create a positive first impression by demonstrating and explicitly discussing their commitment to personal development and reflective practice. Platzer et al. (2000) observed that the socialisation and previous experiences of nurses and the culture in which they work do not always foster the openness that shared learning requires. Joint working between HEIs and placement partners as well as adequate training and updates for mentors can all contribute towards a reflective culture.

Wilkes (2006) carried out a literature review on the student–mentor relationship and highlighted that there is complexity and conflict between the various mentoring roles. She outlined that clear boundaries should be set, expectations made clear and roles and responsibilities defined at the outset. In practice, the mentor and student may use a variety of reflective techniques together. These should be negotiated and an awareness of the issue of power and the mentor's role in assessment considered. Hargreaves (2004) argued that reflection may place individuals in a position of vulnerability and that moral and ethical issues need to be considered when reflection moves to a more public domain. O'Donovan (2005) investigated factors influencing the use of reflection by psychiatric nursing students on placement. She identified that mentors play an important role, but that the level of involvement varied considerably. This appeared to be due to lack of awareness about reflection by mentors and the quality of the relationship, in particular the development of trust being considered key. In order to begin this process, mentors and students are strongly advised to meet either before the placement starts or within the first few days. The points to discuss at a first meeting can be considered under three headings (Sharp *et al.* 2005):

1. Practicalities
2. Building the relationship
3. Background information.

In mentor preparation courses, participants are encouraged to apply Maslow's (1987) Hierarchy of Needs and Knowles' (1990) Adult Learning Theory to ensure that they consider the students' needs, personal and professional experiences and motivations. This contributes to setting the tone of the relationship that then may foster reflective dialogue. Mentors should ascertain the students' previous experiences of reflection, if they keep a diary and, if so, how they would like to use it. Burton (2000) commented that novices of reflection need a suitable tool to develop the skills of synthesis, analysis, critical thinking and evaluation rather than just pontificating or ruminating over an experience. Developing these skills by keeping a narrative diary may prove useful for students (Forneris and Peden-McAlpine 2006). McClure (2002), in an accessible overview of reflection (available online at www.practicebasedlearning.org) described three cases of students who started to keep a diary late in their course and regretted not starting earlier as the benefits were realised; they made comments such as 'it helped me get the day into perspective'. McClure (2002) also noted that it is important to report thoughts, feelings and opinions rather than just factual events and to remember positive experiences and achievements. Further help can be found in Melanie Jasper's chapter about journal keeping (Chapter 7).

Facilitation of learning, the context for practice and evidence-based practice

Prior to starting a placement, a student will have identified his/her own personal learning needs, considered the learning opportunities available and then identified specific learning goals. Greenwood (1998) identified the importance of reflecting before action so that thought is given to what one intends to do and how one intends to do it before actually doing it. An appreciation of the student's learning style or preferences (Kolb and Fry 1975; Honey and Mumford 2000; Fleming 2007) may be of benefit to the mentor in selecting approaches to facilitating learning, and Fleming (2007) has offered some excellent guidance on matching facilitative approaches to learning styles (available at www.vark-learn. com). In some placement areas at Oxford, a small card has been developed that reminds students to reflect on their learning daily. It is two-sided and either laminated or of a bright colour. One version has both Gibbs *et al.* (1988) and Atkins and Murphy's (1993) reflective frameworks on it (E. Burns, unpublished teaching material, Oxford Brookes University, 2007). Another (adapted) version below has a reminder to set goals using SMART criteria (Specific, Measurable, Achievable, Realistic and Time-related) (Renal Ward, Oxford Radcliffe NHS Trust (ORHT)). Students find this card useful each day in order to start the reflective process and recall what they have learned and what they need to develop (see Fig. 4.3).

Bloom's (1956) taxonomy is also useful in helping students and mentors to find the language to set challenging goals or objectives that embrace cognitive, affective and psychomotor domains. Students often need help to progress from broad and task-focused objectives to more specific, holistic and personal goals.

One of the challenges that mentors face is how to facilitate learning in an increasingly busy and pressured environment where they play a vital

Ward/department/placement name:	Today's shift was with:
Main learning objectives/goals for the day: SMART • • • •	• Additional learning achieved today: • Areas for future practice/further development: • Areas of good practice:

Fig. 4.3 Small card for students to use in practice (adapted from Renal Ward (ORHT))

role in helping students to develop reflective skills (Clouder 2000). Initially on a placement, students will progress from observing mentors going about their practice to becoming participants and, increasingly, developing independence. Most learning in practice adopts an experiential approach (Kolb 1984) where an experience is followed by reflection. Clouder (2000) described how following internal and personal reflection, clinicians go on to discuss their work with colleagues engaging in dialogical reflection, usually informally, either before or after practice. This unprompted reflection with others is more likely to occur after a problematic or challenging situation. These practice situations are what Schön (1983) described as the swampy lowlands of practice problems. Johns (2006) realised that just talking through his own reflection with another helps him to explore ideas, and 'listening to himself' helps contradictions become evident.

Loughran (2002) stated that it is not surprising that reflection continually emerges as a way of helping practitioners better understand what they know and do, as they develop their knowledge of practice through reconsidering what they learn in practice. As McClure (2002) noted, the time for reflection should be integral to ways of working. It does not have to occur at a particular time and can be in-between activities, on the way to and from work, or as a final activity at the end of the day. At first, students themselves may not appreciate the potential learning and complexity of practice (Levett-Jones and Bourgeois 2007) and engaging in meaningful dialogue may help this process (Ironside 2006). In a small phenomenological study, O'Donovan (2007) suggested that mental health nurses found that engaging in reflective discussions with preceptors, peers and placement coordinators was constructive and they found it easier than writing reflectively. They saw reflection as a purposeful, thinking activity that heightened their self-awareness and helped to highlight strengths and limitations. Several of the students in O'Donovan's study highlighted changed practice as a result of reflecting. The time to reflect was identified by the students in O'Donovan's study as a problem. It appeared to be easier in areas where it was structured into the day, although some of the students commented that there was a lack of awareness and no culture of reflection in some placements. Therefore students themselves may have a role to play in role-modelling reflection to their mentors and engaging in discussions that show their mentors the benefits of reflective approaches to practice.

Price (2005), as part of a series of supplements on the mentoring role, outlined the benefits of 'thinking aloud your practice' and some practical ways for mentors to develop confidence and competence in a staged way. Tsang (2007) discussed 'reflection as dialogue' in social work practice and described various approaches to developing reflective dialogue as a solitary activity, with colleagues or in teams. She raised the need to consider power relationships and outlined the benefits for broadening perspectives and raising awareness.

Chapter 4

Mentors and students have identified role modelling as an important part of their role (Wiseman 1994; Donaldson and Carter 2005). Bandura (1977) outlined how role modelling is more than imitation and how the behaviour of an individual can be modified by observing the behaviour of another. Donaldson and Carter (2005) found from their focus groups of 42 pre-registration nursing students that they clearly wanted a role model who would allow them to both observe and practise skills or behaviours. They concluded that mentors need to have training on the value of role modelling and how they can further enable students to convert observed behaviour into development of their own skills. This not only applies to clinical and professional skills and behaviours but also approaches to personal learning such as reflection. Therefore, if the benefits and skills of reflection are promoted in all mentor preparation courses and mentors are encouraged to reflect on their own practice in clinical supervision, with their link lecturers/tutors and as part of the reflective dialogue in practice, students will be more likely to use the skills themselves.

Evidence-based practice (EBP) is also considered part of the role of a mentor (NMC 2006) and part of being an effective role model is to demonstrate safe and evidence-based practice (Melnyk 2007). There has been some stimulating debate on the relevance of the traditional hierarchy of evidence (Rolfe 2002), and Mantzoukas (2007) asserted that the evidence-based practice movement may benefit much more from the use of reflection on practice. Importantly, most definitions of EBP (Rycroft-Malone et al. 2004) include the need for professional knowledge and experience to be used alongside research and patient preferences. This professional knowledge can be enhanced when practitioners adopt a reflective approach to their professional development, as discussed earlier.

Reflection also plays a part in the learning and teaching of both professional and clinical skills. There are several frameworks that are valuable in helping mentors to teach clinical skills (Fitts and Posner 1967; Peyton 1998) that seem to equate well to Kolb's (1984) work and recognise the place of reflection and evaluation of learning. Often a structured approach to teaching, demonstrating and practising clinical skills is neglected and frameworks such as these can provide a focus for both the mentor and the student.

Assessment and accountability: evaluation of learning and leadership

Mentors have a clear role in assessing practice and the NMC (2006) has emphasised the importance of accountability, in particular at the point leading to registration, and has identified a new role of 'sign-off mentor'. Work by Duffy (2004a, 2004b) highlighted that practitioners were 'failing to fail' students and she indicated that mentors need an opportunity to

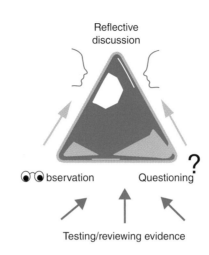

Reflective
discussion

Observation   Questioning

Testing/reviewing evidence

Fig. 4.4   Skills brought together by reflective discussion

reflect with lecturers when they have failed students as it is emotionally draining. There are several references and examples throughout the study that refer to the lack of clear evidence that supports or refutes student competence. Therefore mentors need to ensure they are rigorous in their assessment processes and should reflect on their own performance and development in this key part of their role. Sharp *et al.* (2005) equated the skills that mentors use in assessing students to those they have developed when assessing patients/clients: observation (Shakespeare 2005), questioning (Philips and Duke 2001) and testing/reviewing evidence. These skills are brought together by reflective discussion as illustrated in Fig. 4.4.

Cowan *et al.* (2005) undertook a literature review on competence and recounted the philosophical changes that have occurred in recent years as nurse education has moved from an apprenticeship model to a competency-based approach. They concluded that there is little consensus on what competency is. They surmised that nursing practice requires a combination of knowledge, skills, performance, values and attitudes in a more holistic conception of competence. Fade (2005) has offered several activities for students and their mentors to use on placement as part of the range of resources and learning materials (available at www.practice-basedlearning.org). These include reflective questions, supervisor observation proforma and video clips. Fade also advises how students can start to collate their reflection as evidence for competency achievement. Allin and Turnock (2007) outlined that evidence that demonstrates competence should be carefully selected, personally meaningful and professionally presented.

O'Donovan (2007) described how students write up reflections in their competency booklet as evidence of how and why they think they are competent. Students' reflections are not assessed; rather they are seen as an aid to learning and as a development tool. At Oxford this same process forms part of the student's portfolio. The reflections are used as a basis for reflective discussions, they inform future mentors of developmental progress and the student can develop them into larger reflective pieces if an experience was particularly meaningful. McCready (2007) highlighted the challenges of using portfolios as part of the assessment of competence and recommended clear guidelines for their use.

Once in the public sphere, reflections are open to scrutiny (Cotton 2001) and so may be considered as a source of evidence for practice performance. On reviewing this evidence, mentors may select issues (areas of knowledge or attitude) that warrant further discussion or identify from reflection on skills achievement that the student needs further practice. Cotton (2001) also noted that the views of patients are rarely sought in judging whether a reflective practitioner's care is adequate, yet several reflective frameworks ask for the perspective of others. This involvement of patients in the assessment of students is a potential minefield, but of value where students themselves could incorporate feedback from patients regarding their care. In addition, mentors could talk to patients following student reflection to check out the varying perspectives. This potentially has ethical and validity issues that should be explored by HEIs and placement organisations.

The mentor's role in relation to leadership involves taking responsibility for planning the student's learning experience and liaising with other professions to enhance this learning experience (NMC 2006). Mentors should contribute to audit activities and instigate or implement change in order to improve the student's learning experiences where appropriate. Engagement in audit activity complements reflection-on-practice as it involves a more formal and structured analysis and review of practice. Gould et al. (2007) outlined the implications of the NHS KSF for nursing, and concluded that the core dimension 2 (Personal and People Development) and specific dimension 19 (Leadership) relate well to the NMC (2006) standards.

Conclusion

We have examined the context of practice and its impact on students and mentors. In addition, the place of reflection in practice learning has been discussed. The introduction of the NMC (2006) Standards to Support Learning and Assessment in Practice has been outlined and we have considered how reflection plays an important role in life-long learning and continued professional development. The student's journey into reflection has been explored using some of the practical examples and approaches that we utilise to teach a range of reflective skills. We have examined the mentor's journey into reflection, discussing the mentor preparation course and some of the activities used to introduce or develop reflective skills in mentors.

Disappointingly there are few explicit references to the place of reflection in the mentor's role (NMC 2006) and so the potential for reflective activities on placement has been discussed with examples from our own experiences and related broadly to the eight domains of the standards. Although there has been debate and criticism of reflective practice (e.g. Burnard 2005) we are convinced that reflection has a key role in placement learning; as Loughran (2002, p.33) stated, the reflective practice bandwagon has developed a variety of meanings as it has travelled through the world of practice, but 'has an allure that is seductive in nature because it rings true for most people as something useful and informing'.

References

Allin, L. and Turnock, C. (2007) *Reflection on and in the Workplace*. Available at http://www.practicebasedlearning.org/resources/materials/docs/reflection%20work%20based%20supervisors/index.htm, accessed 27/10/07.

Andrews, M. and Wallis, M. (1999) Mentorship in nursing: a review of the literature. *Journal of Advanced Nursing*, **29** (1), 201–207.

Atkins, S. and Murphy, K. (1993) Reflection: a review of the literature. *Journal of Advanced Nursing*, **18** (8), 1188–1192.

Bandura, A. (1977) *Social Learning Theory*. Prentice-Hall, Englewood Cliffs.

Banning, M. (2004) Approaches to teaching: current opinions and related research. *Nurse Education Today*, **25** (7), 502–508.

Barrows, H. (1986) A taxonomy of problem based learning. *Medical Education*, **20** (6), 481–486.

Bloom, B.S. (ed.) (1956) *Taxonomy of Educational Objectives, the Classification of Educational Goals. Handbook I: Cognitive Domain*. McKay, New York.

Brackenbreg, J. (2004) Issues in reflection and debriefing: how nurse educators structure experiential activities. *Nurse Education in Practice*, **4**, 264–270.

Brookfield, S.D. (2001) *Developing Critical Thinkers: Challenging Adults to Explore Alternative Ways of Thinking and Acting*, 5th edn. Open University Press, Buckingham.

Bulman, C. (2004) Teachers' and students' perspectives on reflection-on-action. In: *Reflective Practice in Nursing* (eds. C. Bulman and S. Schutz), 3rd edn. Blackwell Science, Oxford.

Burnard, P. (2005) Reflections on reflection. *Nurse Education Today*, **25** (2), 85–86.

Burton, A.J. (2000) Reflection: nursing's practice and education panacea? *Journal of Advanced Nursing*, **31** (5), 1009–1015.

Chapple, M. and Aston, E.S. (2004) Practice learning teams: a partnership approach to support students' clinical learning. *Nurse Education in Practice*, **4** (1), 43–49.

Chatterjee, M. (2004) Are skills labs a true training ground? *Nursing Times*, **100** (24), 12–21.

Clouder, L. (2000) Reflective practice – realising its potential. *Physiotherapy*, **86** (10), 517–521.

Clouder, L. and Sellers, J. (2004) Reflective practice and clinical supervision: an inter-professional perspective. *Journal of Advanced Nursing*, **46** (3), 262–269.

Cotton, A.H. (2001) Private thoughts in public spheres: issues in reflection and reflective practices in nursing. *Journal of Advanced Nursing*, **36** (4), 512–519.

Cottrell, S. (2005) *Critical Thinking Skills: Developing Effective Analysis and Argument*. Palgrave Macmillan, New York.

Cowan, D.T., Norman, I. and Coopamah, V.P. (2005) Competence in nursing practice: a controversial concept – a focused review of literature. *Nurse Education Today*, **25** (5), 355–362.

Daloz, L. (1986) *Effective Teaching and Mentoring: Realizing the Transformational Power of Adult Learning Experiences*. Jossey-Bass, San Francisco.

Department of Health (2001) *Working Together, Learning Together: A Framework for Lifelong Learning*. DH, London.

Department of Health (2004) *The NHS Knowledge and Skills Framework*. HMSO, London.

Donaldson, J.H. and Carter, D. (2005) The value of role modelling: perceptions of undergraduate and diploma (adult) nursing students. *Nurse Education in Practice*, **5**, 353–359.

Duffy, K. (2004a) Mentors need more support to fail incompetent students. *British Journal of Nursing*, **13** (10), 582.

Duffy, K. (2004b) *Failing Students*. NMC, London. Available at http://www.nmc-uk.org/aframedisplay.aspx?documentid=1330andkeyword=,accessed 24/10/07.

Edmond, C.B. (2001) A new paradigm for practice education. *Nurse Education Today*, **21**, 251–259.

Elder, L. and Paul, R. (1998) The role of Socratic questioning in thinking, teaching and learning. *The Clearing House*, **71** (5), 297—301. Cited in Harris, M. (2007) Scaffolding reflective journal writing – negotiating power play and position. *Nurse Education Today*, doi:10.1016/j.nedt.2007.06.006.

Fade, S. (2005) *Learning and Assessing Through Reflection*. Available at http://www.practicebasedlearning.org/resources/materials/docs/royalbromptonv3.pdf, accessed 27/10/07.

Fitts, PM. and Possner, M.I. (1967) *Human Performance*. Brookes Cole, Belmont.

Fleming, N. (2007) *VARK: A Guide to Learning Styles*. Available at www.vark-learn.com, accessed 24/10/07.

Forneris, S.G. and Peden-McAlpine, C.J. (2006) Contextual learning: a reflective learning intervention for nursing education. *International Journal of Nursing Education Scholarship*, **3** (1), Article 17. Available at http://www.bepress.com/ijnes/vol3/iss1/art17, accessed 13/11/08.

Fowler, J. (2007) Experiential learning and its facilitation. *Nurse Education Today*, 17 Sept (Epub).

Ghaye, T. and Lillyman, S. (1997) *Learning Journals and Critical Incidents: Reflective Practice for Health Care Professionals*. Mark Allen Publishing, Salisbury.

Chapter 4

Gibbs, G., Farmer, B. and Eastcott, D. (1988) *Learning by Doing. A Guide to Teaching and Learning Methods*, pp. 46–47. FEU, Birmingham Polytechnic.

Gould, D., Berridge, E. and Kelly, D. (2007) The National Health Service Knowledge and Skills Framework and its implications for continuing professional development in nursing. *Nurse Education Today*, **27** (1), 26–34.

Green, C. (2002) Reflecting on reflection: students' evaluation of their moving and handling education. *Nurse Education in Practice*, **2**, 4–12.

Greenwood, J. (1998) The role of reflection in single and double loop learning. *Journal of Advanced Nursing*, **27** (5), 1048–1053.

Hall, W. (2006) Developing clinical placements in times of scarcity. *Nurse Education Today*, **26**, 627–633.

Hargreaves, J. (2004) So how do you feel about that? Assessing reflective practice. *Nurse Education Today*, **24**, 196–201.

Harris, M. (2007) Scaffolding reflective journal writing – negotiating power, play and position. *Nurse Education Today*, doi:10.1016/j.nedt.2007.06.006.

Hilton, P.A. and Pollard, C.L. (2004) Supporting clinical skills development. *Nursing Standard*, **18** (35), 31–36.

Honey, P. and Mumford, A. (2000) *The Learning Styles Questionnaire: 80 Item Version*. Peter Honey Publications, Maidenhead.

Ironside, P.M. (2006) Using interpretive learning and practising interpretive thinking. *Journal of Advanced Nursing*, **55** (4), 478–486.

Jasper, M. (2006) *Professional Development, Reflection and Decision Making*. Blackwell Publishing, Oxford.

Johns, C. (2002) *Guided Reflection: Advancing Practice*. Blackwell Publishing, Oxford.

Johns, C. (2006) *Engaging Reflection in Practice: A Narrative Approach*. Blackwell Publishing, Oxford.

Knowles, M. (1990) *The Adult Learner: A Neglected Species*. Gulf Publishing, Houston.

Kolb, D.A. (1984) *Experiential Learning. Experience as a Source of Learning and Development*. Prentice Hall, New Jersey.

Kolb, D.A. and Fry, R. (1975) Towards an applied theory of experiential learning. In: *Theories of Group Process* (ed. C. Cooper). John Wiley, London.

Levett-Jones, T.L. (2007) Facilitating reflective practice and self-assessment of competence through the use of narratives. *Nurse Education in Practice*, **7**, 112–119.

Levett-Jones, T. and Bourgeois, S. (2007) The clinical placement: an essential guide for nursing students. Cited in Levett-Jones, T. (2007) Facilitating reflective practice and self-assessment of competence through the use of narratives. *Nurse Education in Practice*, **7** (2), 112–119.

Loughran, J.J. (2002) Effective reflective practice: in search of meaning in learning about teaching. *Journal of Teacher Education*, **53** (33), 33–43.

Luft, J. and Ingham, H. (1955) The Johari window, a graphic model of interpersonal awareness. Proceedings of the Western Training Laboratory in Group Development, University of California, Los Angeles. In: Rungapadiachy, D. (1999) *Interpersonal Communication and Psychology for Health Care Professionals*. Butterworth Heinemann, Oxford.

Chapter 4

Maddison, C. (2004) Supporting practitioners in reflective practice. In: *Reflective Practice in Nursing* (eds. C. Bulman and S. Schutz), 3rd edn. Blackwell Science, Oxford.

Magnusson, C., O'Driscoll, M. and Smith, P. (2007) New roles to support practice learning – can they facilitate expansion of placement capacity? *Nurse Education Today*, **27** (6), 643–650.

Mallik, M. and McGowan, B. (2007) Issues in practice based learning in nursing in the United Kingdom and the Republic of Ireland: results from a multi-professional scoping exercise. *Nurse Education Today*, **27**, 52–59.

Mantzoukaz, S. (2007) A review of evidence-based practice, nursing research and reflection: levelling the hierarchy. *Journal of Clinical Nursing* (online early articles). Aailable at http://www.blackwell-synergy.com/doi/abs/10.1111/j.1365-2702.2006.01912.x, accessed 16/10/07.

Maslow, A. (1987) *Motivation and Personality*, 3rd edn. Harper and Row, New York.

McClure, P. (2002) *Reflection on Practice*. Available at http://www.practice-basedlearning.org/resources/materials/docs/reflectiononpractice.pdf, accessed 20/10/07.

McCready, T. (2007) Portfolios and the assessment of competence in nursing: a literature review. *International Journal of Nursing Studies*, **44** (1), 143–151.

McGrath, D. and Higgins, A. (2006) Implementing and evaluating reflective practice group sessions. *Nurse Education in Practice*, **6** (3), 175–181.

McLoughlin, M. and Darvill, A. (2007) Peeling back the layers of learning: a classroom model for problem based learning. *Nurse Education Today*, **27** (4), 271–277.

McMullan, M. (2006) Students' perceptions on the use of portfolios in pre-registration nursing education: a questionnaire survey. *International Journal of Nursing Studies*, **43** (3), 333–343.

Melnyk, B. (2007) The evidence based practice mentor: a promising strategy for implementing and sustaining EBP in health care systems. *Worldviews on Evidence Based Nursing*, **4** (3), 123–125.

Moore, D. and Way, S. (2004) *A report prepared for the Midwifery Committee*. Nursing and Midwifery Council, Pre-Registration Midwifery Education Review Steering Group. Available at www.nmc-uk.org/aframedisplay.aspx?documentid=1166, accessed 25/10/07.

Nursing and Midwifery Council (2004) *Standards of Proficiency for Pre-Registration Nurse Education*. NMC, London.

Nursing and Midwifery Council (2005) *Consultation on Fitness to Practice at the Point of Registration*. NMC, London.

Nursing and Midwifery Council (2006) *Standards to Support Learning and Assessment in Practice. NMC Standards for Mentors, Practice Teachers and Teachers*. NMC, London.

Nursing and Midwifery Council (2007a) *Review of the Code of Conduct*. Available at www.nmc-uk.org, accessed 26/10/07.

Nursing and Midwifery Council (2007b) *Introduction of Essential Skills Clusters for Pre-Registration Nursing Programmes*. Circular 07/07 plus annexe 1 and 2. NMC, London.

O'Donovan, M. (2005) Reflecting during clinical placement – discovering factors that influence pre-registration psychiatric nursing students. *Nurse Education in Practice*, **6** (3), 134–140.

O'Donovan, M. (2007) Implementing reflection: insights from pre-registration mental health students. *Nurse Education Today*, **27** (6), 610–616.

O'Regan, H. and Fawcett, T. (2006) Learning to nurse: reflections on bathing a patient. *Nursing Standard*, **20** (46), 60–64.

Peyton, J. (1998) *Teaching and Learning in Medical Practice*. Manticore Europe, London.

Pfund, R., Dawson, P., Francis, R. and Rees, B. (2003) Learning how to handle emotionally challenging situations: the context of effective reflection. *Nurse Education in Practice*, **4**, 107–113.

Philips, N. and Duke, M. (2001) The questioning skills of clinical teachers and preceptors: a comparative study. *Journal of Advanced Nursing*, **33** (4), 523–549.

Platzer, H., Snelling, J. and Blake, D. (1997) Promoting reflective practitioners in nursing: a review of theoretical models and research into the use of diaries and journals to facilitate reflection. *Teaching in Higher Education*, **2** (2), 103–121.

Platzer, H., Blake, D. and Ashford, D. (2000) An evaluation of the process and outcome of learning through reflective practice groups on a post-registration nursing course. *Journal of Advanced Nursing*, **31** (3), 689–695.

Price, B. (2005) Thinking aloud your practice. *Nursing Standard*, **19** (31).

Quality Assurance Agency (2001) *Code of Practice for the Assurance of Academic Quality and Standards in Higher Education: Section 9 (Placement Learning)*. Available at www.qaa.ac.uk, accessed 24/10/07.

Racey, A. (2005) Using reflective practice as a learning tool in clinical supervision. *Therapy Weekly*, 14 April.

Reid, B. (1993) But we're doing it already. Exploring a response to the concept of reflective practice in order to improve its facilitation. *Nurse Education Today*, **13**, 305–309.

Rolfe, G. (2002) Reflective practice, where now? *Nurse Education in Practice*, **2** (1), 21–29.

Royal College of Nursing (2004) *The Future Nurse: The RCN Vision*. RCN, London.

Rungapadiachy, D. (1999) *Interpersonal Communication and Psychology for Health Care Professionals*. Butterworth Heinemann, Oxford.

Rycroft-Malone, J., Seers, K., Titchen, A., Harvey, G., Kitson, A. and McCormack, B. (2004) What counts as evidence in evidence-based practice? *Journal of Advanced Nursing*, **47** (1), 81–90.

Schön, D. (1983) *The Reflective Practitioner*. Basic Books, London.

Shakespeare, P. (2005) Mentoring and the value of observation. *Nursing Management*, **11** (10), 32–35.

Sharp, P., Ainsley, T., Hemphill, A., *et al.* (2005) *Mentoring: A Resource*. Available at www.practicebasedlearning.org, accessed 34/10/07.

Sully, P. and Dallas, J. (2005) *Essential Communication Skills for Nursing Practice*. Elsevier Mosby, Philadelphia.

Taylor, B. (2006) *Reflective Practice: A Guide for Nurses and Midwives*, 2nd edn. McGraw-Wilson, Maidenhead.

Chapter 4

Tsang, N.M. (2007) Reflection as dialogue. *British Journal of Social Work*, **37**, 681–694.

Turner, D. and Beddoes, L. (2007) Using reflective models to enhance student learning: experiences of staff and students. *Nurse Education in Practice*, **7**, 135–140.

United Kingdom Central Council (1999) *Fitness for Practice*. NMC, London.

Wagner, F. (2007) Vice-President of International Council of Nurses. Key note speech: *Beyond the Borders: International Nursing Education in the 21st Century*. Royal College of Nursing, Brighton.

Watson, S. (2004) Mentor preparation: reasons for undertaking the course and expectations of the candidates. *Nurse Education Today*, **24** (1), 30–40.

Wilkes, Z. (2006) The student mentor relationship: a review of the literature. *Nursing Standard*, **20** (37), 42–47.

Williams, B. (2001) Developing critical reflection for professional practice through problem-based learning. *Journal of Advanced Nursing*, **34** (1), 27–34.

Wilson, M., Shepherd, I., Kelly, C. and Pitzner, J. (2005) Assessment of low fidelity human patient simulator for the acquisition of nursing skills. *Nurse Education Today*, **25**, 56–67.

Wiseman, R.F. (1994) Role model behaviours in clinical setting. *Journal of Nurse Education*, **33** (9), 405–410.

Using reflection in a palliative care education programme

Jane M. Appleton

Introduction

Reflection is widely used in education programmes in the United Kingdom and internationally. In this chapter I want to share my experiences of working as part of a teaching team that has been using reflection in a palliative care programme for more than a decade. In exploring this experience of working with students on their journeys to becoming reflective practitioners I concentrate on two distinct areas. First, I examine some of the challenges inherent in supporting students in this process. Second, I investigate how support strategies may be used when working with students new to reflection. The overall aim of this chapter therefore is to draw on that experience of working with post-qualifying and post-graduate students to nurture their reflective abilities, in order to develop them as reflective practitioners within the context of a palliative care education programme.

Specifically, this chapter has the following aims:

- to explore some of the student and teacher issues involved in using reflection in a post-qualifying and post-graduate palliative care programme;
- to consider strategies for supporting students in the process of developing reflective skills within an education programme;
- to investigate some of the challenges involved in utilising reflection within higher education given the current policy context and pressures facing students, supervisors and tutors.

Reflection as a strategy underpinning the whole curriculum

The reflective approach adopted in the palliative care programme underpinned the entire curriculum and the underlying values of the programme.

It aimed to develop sensitive, responsive, knowledgeable and skilled practitioners who could meet the needs of patients and families with palliative care needs. These values were explicit within the course documentation and were shared by the academic staff delivering the programme. For example, the teaching team modelled reflective skills in their teaching and practice and reflection was used as a teaching method and lived as an underlying philosophy.

As a course tutor and practitioner, I aimed to model and 'live' these values within my teaching, education and palliative care practice in order to be authentic and to demonstrate congruence between my clinical practice and educational activity. The values, beliefs and philosophy underpinning educational activity need to be explicit, transparent and open for debate. The underpinning philosophies of education and palliative care included valuing practice experiences as part of a range of sources of knowledge (Gamble *et al.* 2001), valuing self-awareness and self-directed learning skills, effective communication, patient and family centred care, the client–practitioner relationship and holistic practice in order to enhance the quality of life of patients and families with palliative care needs.

Encouraging the use of reflective diaries from the outset

Several authors have recommended keeping a diary or journal, of some kind, to record practice incidents for reflection (Jasper 1999; Johns 2002). In the palliative care programme students were encouraged to keep a reflective diary throughout the course in order to recall significant events from their practice. It is often difficult to recall the details of practice events after the event; therefore journals are a valuable tool in this process. Burnard (2005) goes further by casting doubt on the ability of students to remember practice events correctly, due to poor memory, and alleges that reflective accounts may be fictionalised. Burnard's criticism is misplaced given that asking if a story is 'true' is not an appropriate question to ask of a narrative account. In terms of memory, diaries helped to avoid the risk of trying to remember what happened and ensured that students had a large repertoire of practice incidents to draw on during a programme of study. These diaries remained private and confidential to each student and were primarily used as a vehicle for developing and liberating incidences from clinical practice that struck the student in some way, in order to return to the event later to explore it in greater depth according to the module being studied. Importantly, students were able to control who, if anyone, saw their reflective diary. In terms of the assessment process, the journals themselves were not seen by assessors. However, extracts from their reflective journals could be used by students and further developed within their reflective writing within a learning contract format. Further debate about assessment of reflection can be found in Chapter 3 of this book. This approach enabled students to have a public and a private account of their reflective writing. Hargreaves (1997) raised an important point about the ethical issues involved when practitioners use details about patients for reflection without the patients being aware of the process. It is important that practitioners and students are aware of the safeguards in terms of these data being anonymous and that patients' identities are protected.

Reflective journals could be kept in a variety of formats including written notes, tape recorded or videoed. The important thing was that it worked for the students and met their needs, was appropriate to their learning style, and was manageable in terms of the time taken to complete. Melanie Jasper, in Chapter 7, challenges educationalists to consider the ethical issue of asking students to keep a reflective diary if you do not do so yourself. I believe that as an educationalist one needs to have experienced the highs and lows of learning to be reflective to fully understand students' concerns and expectations and by extension be able to support them in this process.

How students are introduced to reflection

Reflection and reflective practice were introduced to students and their supervisors together in a preparation study day immediately prior to starting the programme of study. The course values, the assessment process, theoretical aspects of reflection and tips for getting started were covered within these sessions. In addition, written information in the form of module and supervisor handbooks provided further information on reflection and the experience of previous students. Striking the right balance in these sessions between a comprehensive introduction to reflection and not building it up into something 'more than it really is' could be challenging. The key message for students at this stage was: 'Reflection is not an educational panacea, we encourage critical debate about it; however, our experience suggests you and your practice will benefit, so "have a go"'. Students were able to read examples of written reflection from previous students and to hear the experiences of second-year students as they talked about what was useful when they commenced the programme. It was often helpful to have a mixed group of students – those who were new to reflection together with those who had already completed a year – in order to share experiences.

Getting started

Starting reflection can often be difficult and challenging for students. Glaze's (2002) qualitative study explored the experiences of students

developing reflective skills and the stages the students perceived themselves as having gone through in their reflective journeys. Initially, students were described as having 'entry shock' and 'struggles' when they
resisted or were less than positive about the approach. Experience and
research in this area would suggest that reflection is a developmental
process and needs to be learned and worked at over time (Jasper 1999;
Duke and Appleton 2000).

In addition to reflective writing skills, the *depth* of reflective activity
commonly develops over time as students become more confident with
the building blocks of reflective practice. The development of self-awareness as a reflective skill involves students beginning to know themselves
and their practice in an enhanced way. Part of this process is the examination of the student's own assumptions and beliefs about professional
practice and the culture and context of the practice setting. See Sue
Atkins and Sue Schutz's chapter (Chapter 2) for more debate about this
issue.

From my experience, the context of professional practice appears to
have a bearing on the development of reflective skills. For example, in
Africa, where a Diploma in Higher Education in Palliative Care was also
delivered, students tended to be much more aware of the cultural, political and social aspects of palliative care practice. Yet they struggled more
with development of the academic skills, for example, critiquing literature. Conversely, students in the UK were often skilled in the development of critiquing skills, but struggled with the contextual aspects of
practice such as political and social awareness. This may have as much
to do with the availability and access to the academic literature in less
economically developed countries as it has with cultural differences. UK
students commonly only had experience of the NHS, whereas African
students were on the whole more politically and socially aware, probably
due to their need to work across organisations like non-governmental
organisations and faith groups.

Supervision/mentorship

The palliative care programme had been fortunate in being able to
develop highly motivated and skilled supervisors to support students
despite the increased pressures on clinical settings in recent years. Students who had completed the palliative care programme subsequently
became supervisors to other students, building up a pool of skilled and
expert supervisors who had experienced first hand the highs and lows of
learning to reflect. Supervisors were encouraged to engage in critical
debate with students about palliative care practice. They were not
required to grade their student's reflection but were expected to validate
competence in practice. Supervisors were invited to comment alongside

the student's reflective writing to clarify the situation concerned, to question students on their practice story and to attempt to critically debate key issues related to the experience of providing palliative care to patients and families. In addition, supervisors were asked to write their overall comments and evaluate what had gone well and what students needed to work on in subsequent modules. At the end of a module, written feedback was sent directly to supervisors after the assessment process and an opportunity was offered to discuss any development issues with tutors. Supervisors were able to provide evidence of their own learning if they wished to obtain academic credit for a module on teaching and learning.

Wilson et al. (2007), in a research study exploring social work students' experiences of reflecting on their practice, highlighted the importance of the supervisor's role in the development of reflective skills. In particular, they pointed out that the quality of the support and feedback had an impact on the students' reflective abilities, learning from their experiences and their practice. Furthermore, they found that if a positive relationship between students and their supervisors developed, this appeared to have a positive effect on the students' satisfaction and their overall learning, whilst a negative relationship appeared to adversely affect the learning process and to reinforce the students' anxiety.

A number of writers have highlighted the importance of support, supervision and facilitation in the development of reflective writing skills, for example Williams (2000) and Hughes (2007). My experience suggests that the quality of supervision can influence the ability of the student to develop reflective skills, the level of reflection achieved and indeed the overall mark obtained. This raises equity issues in terms of some students having unproblematic access to talented, motivated, experienced supervisors whilst others may not; this could have the effect of compromising learning opportunities for some students.

Students on the programme were able to choose their own supervisors and were encouraged to choose someone they could trust to support them, who they could take challenging feedback from, who had teaching and learning experience consistent with the level at which the student was studying as well as palliative care expertise and knowledge. Additionally, students needed to be able to meet regularly face to face with their supervisors over the course of the module. Whilst face to face meetings were the norm, it is also possible to effectively undertake this process from a distance via email. Whilst the skills required to support students from a distance via email have similarities, there are also differences. For example, students, supervisors and tutors need to spend some time trying to understand the contextual aspects of the practice each are engaged in, in order to learn collaboratively. In addition, supporting students from a distance requires greater clarity in feedback comments and a full and frank discussion prior to commencing the support regarding response times and student and tutor expectations.

Chapter 5

The role of a 'critical friend' has been identified within the literature as an important, some would say essential, part of the reflective process. A critical friend is someone who will listen to and/or read the student's reflection and who will help the student to make sense of his or her practice incidents (Taylor 2006). This relationship, like mentorship, has elements of both support and challenge. A critical friend will be able to listen to the student's practice story and ask key questions to enable the student to analyse the situation in greater depth and to make sense of why this particular practice event or situation has struck him or her. This reflective questioning enables the student to respond (or not) so that ultimately the student remains in charge of the direction of the reflective writing and ownership of the reflection remains with the student. This process requires openness, honesty and trust between a student and supervisor to really enable the relationship to flourish.

Supervisors might act as 'sounding boards' for ideas, occasionally giving an expert viewpoint, supporting a student who is emotionally affected by a practice incident or challenging the student to think through ideas and thoughts so as to stimulate a critical dialogue. A primary function of the supervisor's role is to affirm the student's sense of self-worth while challenging the student to consider alternative perspectives and deepen his/her understanding of the practice situation.

A supervisor's own self-awareness and ability to engage in the process of critical debate is fundamental to his/her ability to support students in the process of developing reflective skills. Supporting supervisors to develop these teaching and learning skills is vitally important within an educational programme utilising reflection. The demands on supervisors in terms of involvement and time to support students in the assessment of competence and reflection in the practice setting can be considerable, given the current contextual pressures in health care. Notwithstanding these demands, the pressures are somewhat dissimilar for pre-registration and post-qualifying programmes. First, within a post-qualifying programme students are experienced practitioners who are often undertaking a programme of study to develop them as specialist and advanced practitioners and do not require the same level of support in practice as pre-registration students. Second, post-qualifying students are commonly in a position to really influence the practice they are engaged in by working with a supervisor to bring about change. In recent years supervisors have been required to observe the students' practice and to validate their competence. This shift further enhances the supervisors' role in that they are in a position to influence practice and to address and bridge the theory–practice gap.

A supervisor in the role of a critical friend needs to be particularly alert to the emotional impact of practice events and be able to help students make sense of their feelings connected with a practice incident. All learning involves an element of risk. Rich and Parker (1995) caution that the process of exploring feelings with students can have a detrimental effect

Box 5.1   Example of the interaction between a tutor and student within a reflective learning contract on a module related to pain management

Tutor comment: *What did you observe in practice? Did you see a range of personal feelings provoked and what sense did you make of this?*

Student's response: I observed a range of feelings in both staff and patients. As well as patients who called him an 'ogre', a passing ambulance driver called him a 'roaring lion' – this echoes the earlier ideas of Nightingale (1914) and Illich (1976) that a person can become treated like an animal. One lady, however, who observed Mr Smith from her chair used to say she felt sorry for him and would question why he was unhappy. Some nurses just told Mr Smith to be quiet and others were apprehensive about seeing to his care needs in case he hit out at them if they hurt his arm. I felt that the noise that Mr Smith made was all that some people were seeing and I am aware that sometimes I just saw the 'noise' because it would impact all over the ward. I think sometimes I saw him as a threat to my professional self, because I was unable to relieve his pain, which is what I felt I should have been able to do. The pain and suffering he experienced seemed to have transformed themselves into the person we saw and it was hard to remember this person had thoughts and feelings like everyone else. The handover of Mr Smith between shifts usually concentrated on how noisy he had been. Reflecting on this now I feel that the outward signs of Mr Smith's suffering were all we could see, somehow blocking out the person experiencing the pain. If Mr Smith perceived that people were not recognising the person behind the suffering then maybe the first adaptive task (Moos and Schaefer 1986) of preserving a satisfactory self-image would have been impossible to attain within that environment.

Tutor comment: *I am left wondering how you coped with this situation in practice and what support you sought from outside the ward team to assist with this difficult pain situation?*

Student's response: Craig (1986) continues that discovering that a setting poses a threat of physical injury can provoke anxiety and avoidant behaviour. Maybe then, when other patients saw Mr Smith not coping with pain, they displayed avoidant behaviour and wanted him nursed in a side room, because they felt their own adaptive behaviour may be personally threatened.

Tutor comment: *Is this what happened? How did staff respond to these requests? What sense did you make of others wanting Mr Smith to be moved out of sight? Might there be some value in other patients and families seeing you do everything possible to support Mr Smith?*

Contd.

Student's response: Staff did try to explain reasons for Mr Smith's behaviour to other patients without disrespecting confidentiality issues. We would always support a patient displaying noisy behaviour like Mr Smith for whatever reason and explain to other patients that he was unwell, did not want or enjoy behaving in that way but could not help it and needed our sympathy, not unkind words. I have noticed the value of explaining this to people and yes, I think they gain some comfort from knowing that Mr Smith is still very much cared about by nursing staff along with his shouting and hitting out. Maybe they are reassured that because staff support and show kindness to Mr Smith despite his behaviour that staff will be equally kind and supportive to other patients' needs. However, when other patients have been kept awake at night, their own needs for rest will always be paramount to them and their families.

on their coping strategies. This concern related to the ethical aspects of learning is not exclusive to reflective learning. However, it may be more likely to occur given the fundamental requirement to explore the feelings provoked within reflective learning. The need for supportive, effective and thoughtful facilitation is paramount. The tripartite nature of the reflective process, of student, supervisor and tutor using a learning contract in the palliative care programme, reduces the likelihood of this happening and provides additional safeguards for students.

Box 5.1 gives an example of the interaction between a tutor and student within a learning contract on a module related to pain management. This specific example was related to an incident in practice when the person's pain was not relieved and how the incident had an impact on the nurse in witnessing the person's distress.

Jasper (1999) has suggested that the ability to take personal, emotional risks in the exploration of practice experiences is fundamental to learning from reflection. Working with students taking risks is commonly a gradual process, dependent on getting to know and trusting one another. This process encourages students to an awareness of why they arrive at a particular decision and enables them to justify and debate their own practice.

One of the most satisfying moments for supervisors and tutors is being witness to perspective transformation (Mezirow 1981), when a student clearly has a changed perspective on his or her practice as a result of reflecting on the experience. This changed perspective might lead to changes in beliefs, attitudes and ultimately alter behaviour in practice. Ferris and von Gunten (2007) suggested that knowledge itself is insufficient to change practice and improve care and that there are sequential

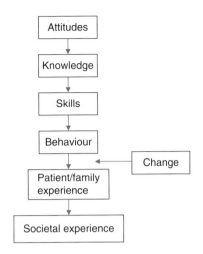

Fig. 5.1   The framework for educational change (Ferris and von Gunten 2007)

steps in the process of educational change (see Fig. 5.1), starting with attitudes and moving to a change in societal experience.

Yet this process of change can be painful and unsettling for students when long-held beliefs and values about their practice are re-assimilated and re-examined in the light of what they have learned. Whilst this can be enlightening and thought provoking for students, it can also be uncomfortable and challenging, and the need for effective support and facilitation is paramount if students are to avoid feeling vulnerable and exposed. The process of examining feelings is not about a confessional approach to exploring practice but more about understanding your own responses to situations.

Experience supporting students in the programme suggests that students' past experience of education, as children or adults, can fundamentally influence their confidence in their own beliefs about their academic ability (Mountford and Rogers 1996; Platzer et al. 2000). I have worked with many mature students who from past educational experience considered themselves to be 'non-academic' and unable to achieve a degree. However, with effective support these students not only achieved this but also flourished in an environment where past experience of both life and practice was highly valued. These negative experiences of education can have a considerable impact on students' self-esteem and their willingness to engage in the process of reflective learning, or, on the other hand, reflection may be an outlet for these past experiences.

In recent years, writers in the nursing literature have been trying to rediscover the emotions once thought of as inappropriate to the nurse/

Chapter 5

patient relationship and to put these back at the centre of the relation-ship (Freshwater and Stickley 2004). Nurses who trained in an era when the exploration of and the attention to feelings was viewed as 'unprofes-sional' may struggle with the concept of reflection and reflective practice, as this can be perceived as not being a legitimate activity or even self-indulgent. The exploration of feelings as part of the reflective process should not leave a student feeling personally exposed. A key issue here is that students retain control of what is disclosed to others and are able to manage how far they take these discussions. There may be a difference between that which is disclosed verbally with supervisors and tutors and that which eventually becomes the reflective assignment. This process embraces both the verbal and written aspects of learning to reflect. In terms of learning, a supervisor will frequently gain as much from the experience of working together as the student who is undertaking the programme; this joint collaborative learning process provides a support-ive platform to explore issues pertinent to practice *together*.

A number of studies have highlighted the potential obstacles to a stu-dent's ability to reflect on his or her practice. These include a lack of ability to analyse situations, a lack of theoretical knowledge, the lack of availability of good supervision and the student's willingness to admit limitations or learning needs (Thompson 2006). The ability to critically analyse situations and develop theoretical knowledge are developmental processes built into a programme of study as part of transferable skills development. However, effective supervision requires supervisor prepa-ration, supervisor confidence, ongoing support and feedback from the teaching team, and skills in self-awareness on the part of the supervisor.

Use of reflective frameworks

A number of authors have suggested the use of frameworks to guide students undertaking reflective writing, especially if the student is new to reflection (Jay and Johnson 2002; Taylor 2006). Johns (2000) has reminded us that models or frameworks for reflection are simply tools to help us rather than a rigid prescriptive format. Jasper (2006) has cau-tioned us that whilst frameworks can be useful, each one comes with the author's particular perspective and values base and leads reflectors in a specific direction. Typically, frameworks have a number of stages and cue questions which enable students to work through a checklist to help structure their reflection. As with any framework, students need to be encouraged to be critical of the model, to ask themselves why a particular framework works for them, or not, and to consider why the author asks the cue questions they do. (See Chapter 9 for further reading about reflective frameworks.)

During the introductory day for the programme, students were intro-duced to a number of frameworks, for example, Gibbs *et al.* (1988), Johns (2000) and Jay and Johnson (2002), and were able to decide which one they found most useful. Many students utilised the reflective cycle (Gibbs *et al.* 1988); the cyclical format and the use of key questions to prompt them in their reflective writing were often effective for new students. These are by no means essential to the process of reflective writing. On the other hand, some authors warn against the use of models and frame-works, suggesting that they could have the effect of stifling creativity in reflective writing and may lead to students being passive and restrained (Bolton 2005). Despite these warnings, at least initially, novice reflectors can benefit from the use of frameworks, enabling them to concentrate on the content of their reflection rather than being overly concerned about the structure.

Feedback and the critical dialogue about practice

In the palliative care programme, reflective writing within a learning con-tract was accompanied by a tripartite critical debate about palliative care practice with a supervisor and tutor. Students' reflective writing was shared with their supervisors and tutors, who were encouraged to respond with reflective questioning and comments. This approach tries to bring together mediated learning (aided by a teacher) and non-mediated learn-ing (experiential) in a way that makes connections between that which students are learning in the programme and their practice experiences. The reflective questioning and comments aim to clarify the situation and the issues that the patient and family are faced with, in order to be able to ask questions of the students' practice to enhance their understanding of palliative care practice and in particular their own practice. These prompts aim to develop the depth of reflection and the students' knowl-edge and skills in palliative care. The challenge for the supervisor and the tutor are to try to move students on to a higher level of reflection. Usually this involves moving from description of a situation and feelings induced by it to critical analysis and evaluation, encouraging students to consider the contextual aspects of practice, for example, the ethical, political, professional and cultural issues involved. (Chapter 9 gives further information on levels of reflection as part of Mezirow's (1981) and Goodman's (1984) frameworks.)

Box 5.2 gives a further example of how this tripartite dialogue, between a student, supervisor and tutor, might look in a module on death and dying. The student's objective is focused on improving her understanding of the essence of spirituality when caring for a person who is dying in a hospice setting.

Box 5.2   An example of how the tripartite reflective dialogue, between a student, supervisor and tutor, might look in a module on death and dying

Student comment: I felt privileged that Eve shared her innermost thoughts with me; it made me feel very close to her. She grabbed on to my hand and I felt she needed human contact, as if it helped her to feel safe. At this moment I felt that a connection had passed between us. She appeared to be very vulnerable and frail and I wanted to protect her. I suppose I felt that way because of being a mother, a woman and a nurse, being in a nurturing role, and when she held my hand it made me feel close to her, an intimate thing and I was allowed into her private space. It made me feel needed and liked. When Eve talked about finding her spirituality, it made me wonder what had happened.

Tutor comment: *You may want to consider internal and external factors at the hospital that made her lose her sense of self and those things you brought to her at the hospice that helped to comfort her and find it again.*

Student comment: Somewhere in the hospital she had lost her spirituality, which made me feel that she had suffered deeply within her; this made me want to protect her from any more harm.

Supervisor comment: *I often feel this way as well, but how can we protect people from suffering and do they really want us to?*

Contd.

Verbal versus written reflection

Some students were skilled at reflecting verbally on their experiences of palliative care practice in an insightful and dynamic way yet found it difficult to transfer this skill to a written format. Johns (2002) highlighted the oral culture of nursing which dominates and privileges speech over writing. This is undoubtedly true if we consider how nurses communicate with each other about patient care in the clinical setting. Students undertaking the degree programme in palliative care needed to be able to function in a range of academic literacies in the current health care environment and so need to be able to function effectively in multiple forms (Lea and Street 2000), reflective writing being just one of these. Furthermore, a student's preferred learning style (Kolb 1984; Honey and Mumford

Student comment: Some older people are vulnerable and are less likely to challenge the authority of health care professionals and less likely to become involved in decision making (Green *et al.* 1994). I think older people often need a much more sensitive approach and they need time to adjust to new decisions. The doctors appeared to be very powerful in their approach and although well meaning in their intentions they made me feel they were acting in a paternalistic way. I know they were trying to balance the well-being and safety of Eve. However, I felt angry because when they stood together they looked powerful, overbearing in fact.

Tutor comment: *Interesting that when you placed yourself alongside the patient, you felt this.*

Student comment: Because I felt the decision was against her wishes, it made me think that the doctors didn't really know her.

Supervisor comment: *Do you think there is a difference between the doctor/patient and the nurse/patient relationship that enables nurses to have more insight into how dying people may want to manage their time left?*

Student comment: Initially I felt that a nurse/patient relationship can foster patients' well-being and is attuned to their individual needs, while doctors are assiduous in trying to solve problems of dysfunction. However, in a study by Lutzen *et al.* (2000) they found that female nurses and physicians experience moral conflicts in their practice to a greater extent than male nurses and physicians, so it may have something to do with gender as to how we communicate with people in general.

2000) will have an impact on his or her propensity to write effectively in a reflective style.

In Chirema's (2007) study exploring the use of reflective journals in promoting reflection and learning in a post-registration nursing programme, some students benefited from journal writing more than others, a number of students preferring to reflect verbally as opposed to the written format. Jasper (1999) highlighted the long-term value of written reflection and discovered that the nurses in her study found that while verbal reflection occurred spontaneously, written reflection was initially difficult and had to be learned, practised and worked at over time. Furthermore, the nurses in this study emphasised that personal attitudes were important and that the commitment of the students to the process of reflective writing was key, i.e. you have got to want to do it.

From my personal experience of working with students who 'get stuck' or who find it difficult to start the process of reflective writing, asking them to tell you the practice narrative verbally and prompting them with reflective questioning can enable them to progress to the written format.

From description to critical analysis

In working with students new to reflective writing who are in the process of developing skills, written reflection is commonly descriptive in nature. It is usual for students to begin in the descriptive domain and it can take time and facilitation for them to develop analytical and critical thinking skills. These students may spend much of the word allowance of an assignment describing what happened and how they felt about the situation. These students generally need to tell their practice story first, sometimes at length and in full before they are able to progress to critically analysing the situation. In an academic assignment, this process is hindered by the inevitable word limit and the restrictions this imposes. The development of reflective skills is intimately associated with the development of critical thinking skills and is one of the ways in which practitioners make sense of their practice and their decision making. Critical thinking skills, according to Jasper (2006, p.103) consist of four subcategories:

- exploring issues;
- making connections;
- organising thoughts/structures;
- taking a new perspective on issues.

Tutors and supervisors have a key role in modelling these critical thinking skills in students by critiquing their own educational and clinical practice and by encouraging students to challenge ideas both in the classroom and within reflective writing.

Assessing reflection

Assessing reflection within an education programme is not a straightforward process; it remains a contentious area despite the increase in published literature in this area (see Chapter 3 for much more detail on this). The outcome of reflective learning can be complicated to measure and demonstrate, given the intangible nature of reflective learning at the end of a programme of study. The key outcome of reflective learning is to demonstrate the impact on the student's practice and ultimately improvement in practice for patients and families (see the framework for educational change above). Specifically, this might be the demonstration of new or enhanced knowledge, the acquisition of new or advanced skills or altered attitudes resulting in a changed behaviour in practice. Providing clarity about exactly what is being assessed is therefore important; this in itself is challenging given that there is no agreement on the definition of reflection. Also there is currently no widely accepted method of assessing reflection (Stewart and Richardson 2000; Watson 2002). Despite this the palliative care programme team created a reflective marking grid, developed from the literature on levels of reflection and framed using the reflective cycle (see Table 5.1). This grid has been refined and adjusted over the years according to university drivers and in line with our increasing experience of assessing reflection. For example, not all categories of the grid were necessarily equally weighted as we knew that contextual issues affecting practice generally take longer to develop and are associated with higher levels of reflection than the ability to describe the event or associated feelings.

A joint approach between a supervisor in clinical practice assessing competence and the teaching team enabled students to be assessed using this grid. Essentially, within an educational programme there needs to be explicit matching of the learning outcomes, assessment tasks and assessment criteria. In feedback from assessments students were given written comments throughout their learning contracts and a copy of the marking grid denoting where they had been marked in relation to each section of the grid. Potentially, this approach requires congruency between the students' performance in practice and their reflective writing skills. One of the key challenges in the evaluation of reflection is how to measure the outcomes of reflective practice from a patient or family's perspective. This is an area of research that is yet to be fully investigated.

The debate concerning the pros and cons of assessing reflection has been well covered by Hargreaves (2004), Schutz et al. (2004) and also by Sue Schutz in Chapter 3 of this book. In essence, Hargreaves argued that a student's desire to do well academically inhibits him or her from reflecting honestly and openly on practice. Additionally, Hargreaves has alleged that there are only three narratives of professional practice which are legitimate, and identifies these as 'valedictory', 'condemnatory' and 'redemptive'. A valedictory narrative, according to Hargreaves, presents a situation in which the practitioner is faced with a difficult decision and ultimately improves the situation. There is a problem or a crisis in practice and the practitioner recognises the problem and turns the situation around. In contrast, a condemnatory narrative presents a situation where there is no resolution, or the outcome is negative. The practitioner feels guilt and/or anger at not being able to resolve the situation. Redemptive narratives, on the other hand, enable students to 'express inappropriate attitudes' so long as these attitudes are 'redeemed' (Hargreaves 2004).

I would challenge Hargreaves' belief that these are the only types of narratives that are legitimate in terms of professional practice, and the

Chapter 5

Table 5.1   The reflective marking grid. Marking criteria for reflective evidence – level 3 (palliative care programme) (with kind permission of Oxford Brookes University)

Grade	A (100%–70%)	B+ (69%–60%)	B (59%–50%)
Ability to set realistic objectives relevant to the module focus	Considerable ability to link objectives with module learning outcomes and personal and professional knowledge of health care practice	Clear ability to link and integrate objectives with module learning outcomes and personal and professional knowledge of health care practice	Moderate ability to link objectives and learning outcomes and personal and professional knowledge of health care practice
Ability to describe the event/situation	Description succinctly captures the essence of the event/situation	Description clearly expressed, on the whole concise and succinct	Description expressed clearly but with some unnecessary detail included
Ability to identify and focus on salient issues from the situation	Description of the event/ situation leads to a clear, concise focus that is consistently followed within the account	Description of the event/ situation leads to a clear focus that is followed within the account	Description of the event/ situation leads to a focus that is mostly followed in the account
Ability to analyse own and others feelings	Demonstrates considerable ability to analyse own and others' feelings carefully, considering alternative perspectives	Demonstrates an ability to analyse own and others' feelings and consideration of alternative perspectives	Demonstrates an ability to analyse own and others' feelings, raising alternative perspectives

C (49%–41%)	D (40%)	Refer (39%–30%)	Fail (30%–0%)
Limited ability to link objectives and learning outcomes and personal and professional knowledge of health care practice	Ability to link objectives and learning outcomes and personal and professional knowledge of health care practice is unclear	Link between objectives, module learning outcomes and personal and professional knowledge of health care practice is extremely tenuous	Link between objectives, module learning outcomes and personal and professional knowledge of health care practice is absent
Description mostly clearly expressed but with some unnecessary detail included	Description lacks focus and includes much unnecessary detail	Description is unfocused and includes much unnecessary detail	Description of the event lacks focus and is unclear
Description of the event/ situation suggests a focus that is partly followed in the account. The account addresses issues that are relevant to the event/situation	Description of the event/ situation suggests a focus. The account addresses issues that are not necessarily relevant to the event/situation or focus	Description of the event/ situation does not lead to an identification of a focus or the issues explored within the account are not relevant to the event/situation	Description of the event/ situation does not lead to a clear focus and the issues explored are not relevant
Some attempt at analysing own and others' feelings and some consideration of alternative perspectives	Limited description of own and others feelings, limited consideration of alternative perspective	Little or no description of feelings of self or others involved in the event/situation	No description of feelings of self or others involved in the event/situation

Contd.

Table 5.1   Contd.

Grade	A (100%–70%)	B+ (69%–60%)	B (59%–50%)
Ability to access and use knowledge from a variety of sources	Locates and accesses a comprehensive and extensive range of relevant sources of information. Evaluates and appraises reliability of sources of information	Locates and accesses an extensive range of relevant sources of information. Appraises reliability of sources of information	Locates and accesses an adequate range of relevant sources of information. Some appraisal of sources of information
Ability to integrate theory and practice	Theory and practice are fully integrated, showing insight, creativity and originality	Theory and practice are clearly integrated	Integration of theory and practice is evident
Ability to analyse the contextual issues	Critical discussion of relevant social, political, cultural, ethical or professional issues	Explores relevant social, political, cultural, ethical or professional issues	Consideration of social, political, cultural, ethical or professional issues
Ability to analyse issues pertinent to inclusion and diversity	Principles of diversity and inclusion are evident throughout own practice. Analysis of potential for discrimination within the situation is incorporated	Principles of diversity and inclusion are evident throughout own practice	Demonstrates appreciation of principles of diversity and inclusion in own practice

C (49%–41%)	D (40%)	Refer (39%–30%)	Fail (30%–0%)
Locates and accesses a limited range of relevant sources of information. Limited evidence of appraisal of sources of information	Locates and accesses a very limited range of sources of information. Very limited appraisal of the sources of information	Locates and accesses an irrelevant/ insufficient range of sources of information. No evidence of appraisal of sources of information	No evidence of locating and accessing sources of information
Integration of theory and practice is limited	Integration of theory and practice is very limited	Insufficient integration of theory and practice	No integration of theory and practice
Some consideration of relevant social, political, cultural, ethical or professional issues	Very limited consideration of relevant social, political, cultural, ethical or professional issues	Insufficient consideration of relevant social, political, cultural, ethical or professional issues	Little or no consideration of relevant social, political, cultural, ethical or professional issues
Shows limited appreciation of principles of diversity and inclusion, but no evidence of active discrimination	Little or no appreciation of the principles of diversity and inclusion. However, no evidence of active discrimination	Explicit discrimination evident in practice or analysis of practice	Explicit discrimination evident in practice

Contd.

Table 5.1   Contd.

Grade	A (100%–70%)	B+ (69%–60%)	B (59%–50%)
Ability to draw together and summarise analysis in order to present a new perspective or revision an existing perspective (synthesis)	Key issues from the analysis are consistently drawn together with exceptional clarity, perception and creativity. Clear indication that the account has led to a new perspective or a revisioning and a deeper understanding	Key issues from the analysis are consistently drawn together with clarity, perception and attempts at creativity. Indication that the account has led to a new perspective or a revisioning and deeper understanding	Key issues from the analysis are drawn together. Indication that the account has led to a new perspective
Ability to identify and discuss the implications for practice which arise from the analysis and synthesis and to summarise learning	Clearly and creatively identifies and discusses the implications for practice which arise from analysis and synthesis. Learning achieved and learning needs identified accurately and perceptively	Clearly identifies and discusses the implications for practice which arise from the analysis and synthesis. Learning achieved and learning needs identified accurately	Identifies and discusses some implications for practice which arise from analysis and synthesis. Some attempt to identify learning achieved and/or learning needs
Ability to draw up an achievable action plan based on the implications raised (action planning)	Succinctly outlines a realistic action plan which addresses the practice implications and the learning needs identified	Outlines a realistic action plan which addresses the practice implications and the learning needs identified	Partly outlines an action plan which addresses the practice implications and the learning needs identified
Writing skills and presentation	Work is own and creative in approach	Work is own and there are attempts at creativity	Work is own and there is evidence of some creativity

C (49%–41%)	D (40%)	Refer (39%–30%)	Fail (30%–0%)
Key issues from the reflection are drawn together in a limited way. Indication that the account has led to a new perspective	Key issues from the reflection are drawn together in a very limited way. Little indication that the account has led to a new perspective	Key issues from the reflection are drawn together tenuously or not at all. No indication that the account has led to a new perspective	Key issues from the reflection are not drawn together. No indication that the account has led to a new perspective
Identifies some implications for practice, which arise from the analysis and synthesis, but discussion of these limited. Some attempt to identify learning achieved and/ or learning needs	Very limited discussion of the implications for practice which arise out of the reflection. Little attempt to identify learning achieved and/ or learning needs	Little or no implication for practice addressed. Little or no attempt to identify learning achieved and/or learning needs	No implication for practice addressed. No attempt to identify learning achieved and/or learning needs
Some attempt to outline a realistic action plan which addresses the practice implication and the learning needs identified	Very limited attempt to outline a realistic action plan which addresses the practice implications and the learning needs identified	Little or no plan of action identified to address either the practice implications or own learning needs	No plan of action identified to address either the practice implications or own learning needs
Work is own but lacks creativity	Work is own but no attempt at creativity	Work is not own and lacks creativity	Work is not own

Contd.

Table 5.1   Contd.

Grade	A (100%–70%)	B+ (69%–60%)	B (59%–50%)
	Structure is logical	Structure is logical	Structure is evident and logical
	Grammar, spelling and punctuation are accurate throughout	Grammar, spelling and punctuation are essentially accurate	Grammar, spelling and punctuation are mostly accurate, but some errors are noted
	Harvard referencing systematic, correct and consistent throughout	Harvard referencing mostly correct and consistent throughout	Harvard referencing is mostly correct; however, some errors are noted
	Professional and academic terminology utilised appropriately in context	Professional and academic terminology mainly utilised appropriately in context	Professional and academic terminology occasionally utilised appropriately in context
	Overall presentation (legibility/visual impact/ delivery) is excellent	Overall presentation (legibility/visual impact/ delivery) is very good	Overall presentation (legibility/visual impact/ delivery) is good
Ability to be an independent learner and to self-evaluate work	Is independent in own learning and is perceptive and accurate in self-evaluation	Usually takes responsibility for own learning and is accurate and insightful in self-evaluation	Is able to take responsibility for own learning and shows some insight in self-evaluation
Professional practice skills (PPS) Identification of PPS achieved within this assignment Signed			

C (49%–41%)	D (40%)	Refer (39%–30%)	Fail (30%–0%)
Structure is implicit	Structure is not apparent	Structure is absent; may lack an introduction or conclusion	Structure is absent
Grammar, spelling and punctuation have several errors	Grammar, spelling and punctuation have many errors which detract from the quality of the work	Grammar, spelling and punctuation are poor with many errors	Grammar, spelling and punctuation are poor with many errors throughout the assignment
Harvard referencing errors are evident	Harvard referencing is incorrect and inconsistent	Harvard referencing is incorrect and inconsistent or absent	Harvard referencing is absent
Professional and academic terminology rarely used appropriately in context	Professional and academic terminology poor throughout	Professional and academic terminology not utilised appropriately or in context	Professional and academic terminology not utilised
Overall presentation (legibility/visual impact/ delivery) is satisfactory	Overall presentation (legibility/visual impact/ delivery) requires greater care	Overall presentation (legibility/visual impact/delivery) detracts from the product of the work	Overall presentation (legibility/visual impact/delivery) is poor
Some evidence of taking responsibility for own learning and includes limited self-evaluation	Little evidence of taking responsibility for own learning; self-evaluation is superficial or absent	Little or no evidence of taking responsibility for own learning; self-evaluation is absent or misconstrued	No evidence of taking responsibility for own learning; self-evaluation is absent

Chapter 5

notion that within the spectrum of safe professional practice there is not room for a wide range of beliefs and values. Indeed, the example given by Hargreaves of a student not wishing to work with a particular client group and writing about this in a reflective assignment strikes me as valuable learning, especially in a pre-registration programme. What we identify as acceptable and unacceptable practice is not so difficult to define in terms of the assessment of reflection. We need to be able to agree safe and unsafe practice. However, within safe practice we should expect a range of attitudes amongst students. This diversity is to be embraced rather than assuming that attitudes can be uniform within the profession.

From my experience of working with students, some struggle with the idea of a learning contract with reflective evidence being demonstrated progressively, so that the assignment itself will be dynamic and evolving with comments and responses throughout rather than a finished, polished document like an essay. These students want their work to be 'neat and tidy' and to be able to see the end of the process or completion rather than an ongoing cycle of learning. Potentially this has a direct resonance for palliative care nursing practice itself, when the 'messiness' and complexities of practice are challenging and difficult to cope with.

The appropriateness of reflection within palliative care education

The use of reflection within a palliative care programme is a particularly appropriate learning tool, given the emotional impact of caring for patients and families with life-threatening illnesses and the 'desire' to develop practitioners who are self-aware and emotionally intelligent. There are now a number of recently published examples of research studies into the use of reflection within palliative care education programmes, both in the UK and internationally, focusing on both nursing and medical education (Taylor et al. 2002; Landmark et al. 2004a, 2004b; Read and Spall 2005).

For example, Landmark et al.'s (2004a) study explored the use of reflective group supervision in a post-graduate palliative care education programme in Norway. This study considered the use of reflection and 'dynamic dialogue' with a group of students within a supervision session over a 2-year period. Students in this study evaluated the reflective supervision sessions within the programme as helping them to develop their theoretical and personal knowledge, and their self-awareness, and they felt supported in their development of insights into palliative care practice.

University educational drivers

The current drivers and pressures within university education within the UK put considerable tensions on supervisors and tutors in their attempts to nurture and support the development of reflective skills in students. Significantly these include the drive to reduce formal assessment loads on students, to increase student numbers within programmes, and to widen the participation of students traditionally excluded from higher education, and the continuing pressures within the National Health Service to release students to attend education programmes, which all increase the demands on those attempting to support students to become critical thinkers and reflective practitioners.

Undoubtedly, using reflection in a palliative care programme, as described above, involves patience and determination to support students in the development of reflective skills and time to nurture their reflective abilities. We have recently seen a shifting emphasis within the higher education sector, making it increasingly difficult to continue with a reflective model in the current climate. Those of us who have experienced the transformative effect of reflection on a student's practice need to consider innovative ways to incorporate the reflective model into our education and practice and to fight for the things that are important in education and health care practice.

Conclusion

This chapter has considered the use of reflection within a post-qualifying and post-graduate palliative care education programme and some of the challenges and opportunities presented by this approach. Reflection as an educational strategy presents practitioners and educationalists with an opportunity to support collaborative learning and to develop skills to enhance students' abilities to engage in critical debate about palliative care practice. The role of the supervisor is particularly significant in supporting and facilitating the reflective process. By acquiring these fundamental skills in the process of reflection, students can enhance their understanding of practice. I have explored some of the issues that enhance and facilitate reflection and reflective practice and conversely some of the issues that provide additional challenges for educators, particularly in the current health care climate.

Acknowledgements

This chapter owes much to the insights gained from sharing with students I have worked with on the diploma, degree and post-graduate programmes in Palliative Care at Oxford Brookes University. I am grateful to the students and mentors who over many years challenged my thinking. In particular, I would like to thank former students Carol Walsh and Sue Cunningham and their supervisors, who generously agreed for me to include extracts from their reflective writing within this chapter. Thanks also to Oxford Brookes University for kind permission to publish Table 5.1, the reflective marking grid (level 3).

References

Bolton, G. (2005) *Reflective Practice – Writing and Professional Development,* 2nd edn. Sage, London.

Burnard, P. (2005) Reflections on reflection. *Nurse Education Today,* **25**, 85–86.

Chirema, K.D. (2007) The use of reflective journals in the promotion of reflection and learning in post-registration nursing students. *Nurse Education Today,* **27**, 192–202.

Duke, S. and Appleton, J. (2000) The use of reflection in a palliative care programme: a quantitative study of reflective skills over an academic year. *Journal of Advanced Nursing,* **32** (6), 1557–1568.

Ferris, F.D. and von Gunten, C.F. (2007) North America. In: *Education in Palliative Care: Building a Culture of Learning* (eds B. Wee and N. Hughes), Chapter 10. Oxford University Press, Oxford.

Freshwater, D. and Stickley, T. (2004) The heart of the art: emotional intelligence in nurse education. *Nursing Inquiry,* **11** (2), 91–98.

Gamble, J., Chan, P. and Davey, H. (2001) Reflection as a tool for developing professional practice knowledge and expertise. In: *Practice Knowledge and Expertise in the Health Professions* (eds J. Higg and A. Titchen), Chapter 15. Butterworth/Heinemann, Oxford.

Gibbs, G., Farmer, B. and Eastcott, D. (1988) *Learning by Doing. A Guide to Teaching and Learning Methods.* FEU, Birmingham Polytechnic.

Glaze, J.E. (2002) Stages in coming to terms with reflection: student advanced nurse practitioners' perception of their reflexive journeys. *Journal of Advanced Nursing,* **37** (3), 265–272.

Goodman, J. (1984) Reflection and teacher education: a case study and theoretical analysis. *Interchange,* **15** (3), 9–26.

Hargreaves, J. (1997) Using patients: exploring the ethical dimension of reflective practice in nurse education. *Journal of Advanced Nursing,* **25**, 223–228.

Hargreaves, J. (2004) So how do you feel about that? Assessing reflective practice. *Nurse Education Today,* **24** (3), 196–201.

Honey, P. and Mumford, A. (2000) *The Learning Styles Questionnaire.* Peter Honey, Maidenhead.

Hughes, N. (2007) Reflective learning. In: *Education in Palliative Care: Building a Culture of Learning* (eds B. Wee and N. Hughes), Chapter 15. Oxford University Press, Oxford.

Jasper, M. (1999) Nurses' perceptions of the value of written reflection. *Nurse Education Today,* **19**, 452–463.

Jasper, M. (2006) *Professional Development, Reflection and Decision-Making.* Blackwell Publishing, Oxford.

Jay, J.K. and Johnson, K.L. (2002) Capturing complexity: a typology of reflective practice for teacher education. *Teaching and Teacher Education,* **18**, 73–85.

Johns, C. (2000) *Becoming a Reflective Practitioner. A Reflective and Holistic Approach to Clinical Nursing, Practice Development and Clinical Supervision.* Blackwell Science, Oxford.

Johns, C. (2002) *Guided Reflection: Advancing Practice.* Blackwell Science, Oxford.

Kolb, D.A. (1984) *Experiential Learning – Experience as a Source of Learning and Development.* Prentice Hall, New Jersey.

Landmark, B., Wahl, A.K. and Bohler, A. (2004a) Group supervision to support competency development in palliative care in Norway. *International Journal of Palliative Nursing,* **10** (11), 542–548.

Landmark, B., Wahl, A.K. and Bohler, A. (2004b) Competence development in palliative care in Norway: a description and evaluation of a postgraduate education programme in palliative care in Drammen, Norway. *Palliative and Supportive Care,* **2** (2), 157–162.

Lea, M.R. and Street, B.V. (2000) Student writing and staff feedback in higher education: an academic literacies approach. In: *Student Writing in Higher Education* (eds M.R. Lea and B.V. Street). Society for Research into Higher Education/Open University Press, London

Mezirow, J. (1981) A critical theory of adult learning and adult education. *Adult Education,* **32**, 3–24.

Mountford, B. and Rogers, L. (1996) Using individual and group reflection in and on assessment as a tool for effective learning. *Journal of Advanced Nursing,* **24**, 1127–1134.

Platzer, H., Blake, D. and Ashford, D. (2000) Barriers to learning from reflection: a study of the use of group work with post-registration students. *Journal of Advanced Nursing,* **31** (5), 1001–1008.

Read, S. and Spall, B. (2005) Reflecting on patient and carer biographies in palliative care education. *Nurse Education in Practice,* **5** (3), 136–143.

Rich, A. and Parker, D.L. (1995) Reflection and critical incident analysis: ethical and moral implications of their use within nursing and midwifery education. *Journal of Advanced Nursing,* **22**, 1050–1057.

Schutz, S., Angrove, C. and Sharp, P. (2004) Assessing and evaluating reflection. In: *Reflective Practice in Nursing* (eds C. Bulman and S. Schutz), 3rd edn, pp. 47–72. Blackwell Publishing, Oxford.

Stewart, S. and Richardson, B. (2000) Reflection and its place in the curriculum: should it be assessed? *Assessment and Evaluation in Higher Education,* **25** (4), 369–380.

Taylor, B.J. (2006) *Reflective Practice: A Guide for Nurses and Midwives,* 2nd edn. Open University Press, Maidenhead.

Taylor, B.J., Bulmer, B., Hill, L., Luxford, C., McFarlane, J. and Stirling, K. (2002) Exploring idealism in palliative nursing care through reflective and action research. *International Journal of Palliative Nursing,* **8** (7), 324–330.

Thompson, N. (2006) *Promoting Workplace Learning.* Policy Press, Bristol.

Chapter 5

Watson, S. (2002) The use of reflection in the assessment of practice. Can you mark learning contracts? *Nurse Education in Practice*, **2**, 150–159.

Williams, B. (2000) Collage work as a medium for guided reflection in the clinical supervision relationship. *Nurse Education Today*, **20** (4), 273–278.

Wilson, G., Walsh, T. and Kirby, M. (2007) Reflective practice and workplace learning: the experience of MSW students. *Reflective Practice*, **8** (1), 1–15.

Using group approaches to underpin reflection, supervision and learning

Bernie Carter and Elizabeth Walker

Introduction

Reflective groups have a huge potential to help nurses reflect on their everyday practice, regardless of whether that practice is in the clinical, management or education arena. Groups offer benefits to nurses working with patients across the whole age spectrum, across the diversity of practice and across the range of arenas in which nursing care is given. Whilst group reflection can bring substantial benefits to the group members and to their care and work, it is by no means a simple solution. If groups have the potential to develop skills, knowledge and capacity, to challenge practice, to be emancipatory and empowering, they equally have the potential to go wrong. Where effective groups may result in energising and enthusing members; ineffective groups may simply fizzle away. Perhaps, more worryingly, ineffective groups may be damaging to morale and result in a 'there's no point in trying' attitude.

In this chapter, group work is explored in terms of some of the wider changes that are occurring in the context of professional learning through reflection. Group reflection and supervision are considered as practices in relation to one-to-one approaches to reflection and supervision. Group work is also examined in terms of the 'good, the bad and the ugly' factors that need to be considered to help ensure that groups are supportive, challenging and helpful to group members. We draw on and reflect upon our own experience of working with groups and weave these experiences in with the established literature.

Learning where you are working

Using groups to develop work-related skills and knowledge is not new and groups exist as part of everyday practice in many practice settings. In recent years the potential for harnessing the 'situated learning' that occurs in 'communities of practice' (Wenger 2000; Lathlean and Le May

2002) has been recognised and there has been a commensurate shift to capitalise and make more explicit the learning that occurs in groups. Abma (2007, p.199) emphasises the way in which situated learning is context-bound in relationships between people and that this 'implies an intimate connection between knowledge and action'. Group work can support this contextual connection for practitioners. Certainly this connectivity is an aspect that we wish to encourage as part of our own reflective group work.

Work-based learning

The acceptance that there is a connection between the setting and the context in which learning takes place underpins, to a greater or lesser degree, the recent interest in both work-based learning (WBL) and the notion of learning organisations. Although Burton (2004, p.199) notes that learning in the workplace 'happens anyway', he further states that 'work based learning is only useful if it is both vital and rigorous' (Burton 2004, p.200). Although learning may well happen anyway, there is increased understanding that 'recognising knowledge gained at work helps empower and liberate individuals' (Brennan and Little 2007, p.6). Flanagan et al. (2000, p.363) highlight the benefits of, and complexities associated with, ensuring that work-based learning actually does work. They note that work-based learning 'takes a structured and learner-managed approach to maximising opportunities for learning and professional development in the workplace' and they further state that the essence of WBL is the 'bringing together of self-knowledge, expertise at work and university knowledge'. Work-based learning can be effective for professionals at different stages of their learning (see, for example, Brown et al. 2007), although Dewar and Walker (1999) note that there can be dissonance between the educational philosophy of work-based learning and how it is actually delivered.

Organisational learning

Organisational learning, regardless of how attractive it may seem to be, is complex, and Gherardi (2001) tackles some of the inherent biases and assumptions within the literature on organisational learning that she believes need to be considered. For example, she states that learning

> '. . . is assumed to be synonymous with change: if a significant change is produced, learning has taken place. However this ignores the fact that many organisational changes occur without any learning taking place, and – vice versa – that learning processes may not give rise to change' (Gherardi 2001, p.131).

Learning organisations

Whilst work-based learning and situated learning can occur as pockets of activity within an organisation, the notion of learning organisations extends the activity throughout the organisation. Although there are many different definitions of what a learning organisation is, Armstrong and Foley (2003, p.75) propose a comprehensive definition. They state that a

> 'learning organisation has appropriate "cultural facets" (vision, values, assumptions and behaviours) that support a learning environment; processes that foster people's learning and development by identifying their learning needs and facilitating their learning; and "structural facets" that enable learning activities to be supported and implemented in the workplace'.

These activities often occur in groups where reflection is an important component.

Why use groups to support reflection, learning and supervision?

Within each of the described approaches (situated learning, work-based learning and learning organisations) there is a move to capitalise on the learning that occurs in groups and teams – particularly within the work-setting – and to make such learning more explicit and valued. Developing professional expertise and knowledge through group reflection and supervision can occur within either the practice setting (embedded as part of practice) or an academic setting (embedded within modules and other learning opportunities). Heiskanen (2007, p.370) notes that increasingly 'expert knowledge is seen as shared, distributed and contextualised' and this can be supported through the use of group work in nursing.

Types of reflective groups

Groups range from very informal groups to ones that are more structured and purposive (e.g., some action learning sets, ALS), to other less structured, more democratic, equitable and co-operative groups. Whilst most of these groups meet face-to-face in the real world there is also potential in exploiting the benefits of newer technologies such as web conferencing, and synchronous and asynchronous e-reflection groups. There is huge potential capacity for on-line groups to extend communities of practice within nursing across geographical, cultural, political and social borders. Kelly *et al.* (2005, p.17) report on an on-line gerontological 'nursing "community of practice" ' which was convened to develop best practice; this community of practice had positive outcomes for the members. Although e-groups offer considerable advantages in terms of extending communities of practice, they still rely on people relating to each other. Social relations are every bit as important in cyberspace groups as real-world groups. Our experience shows that encouraging these relational links to be made, for example through initial introductions and on-going inquiries about the members as individuals rather than disembodied contributors of text, is crucial to effective e-groups. Lee-Baldwin (2005, p.108) also notes, in her study on asynchronous discussion forums (ADFs) with pre-service teachers, that 'social dynamics within groups play an important role in facilitating cognitively in depth levels of reflective thinking' within an ADF.

Rolfe *et al.* (2001) noted that, initially, some people viewed groups with a degree of scepticism and saw them simply as a cost-cutting exercise. Although costs may be contained with group approaches (see White and Winstanley 2006) costs still exist; Rolfe *et al.* (2001) observe that costs are incurred as effective groups require skilled facilitation and facilitators require supervision. Groups are different to, but no less resource-intensive than, other approaches to reflection and supervision. Although group work is now used extensively within nursing (across different settings, specialties and for a range of different purposes) one of its primary functions is to develop the capability and/or competence of the participants through reflection. Often the purpose is seen in terms of not only what the reflection/supervision can do for the person but also what it can do in terms of productivity and other benefits for the organisation. There are many examples of this reciprocation of benefit in the literature. In Alleyne and Jumaa's (2007, p.230) study they used 'a process of executive co-coaching for focused group clinical supervision sessions' with the aim of 'building the capacity for evidence-based clinical nursing leadership'. Thus in this particular example, group clinical supervision was being used as a 'focus for the development of actionable knowledge' (Alleyne and Jumaa 2007, p.235). Clinical supervision within groups is firmly embedded as a practice and there is now a more extensive literature which explores the benefits and disadvantages of it as an approach. Lindgren *et al.* (2005), for example, discuss its use within pre-registration training, whereas other authors have explored its value for hospice nurses (Jones 2003, 2006) and its use within intensive care settings (Lindahl and Norberg 2002).

Action learning sets

Action learning sets (ALS), a style of group working (Mumford 1996), have gained in popularity in nursing, and Douglas and Machin (2004) discuss their value in interdisciplinary collaborative working. ALS provide the setting in which learners seek solutions though a 'cycle of identifying and implementing courses of action, monitoring the results, refining the action, testing again . . .' (Stark 2006, p.24). They have been adopted within nursing in education and practice settings for developing clinical leadership skills (Cunningham and Kitson 2000; Hardacre and Keep 2003), management skills (Booth *et al.* 2003), nursing practice (Garbett *et al.* 2007; Hardy *et al.* 2007), enhancing patient safety (Court 2003) and implementing the Modern Matron (Dealey *et al.* 2007). Our experience covers using ALS within developing the supervisory competence of higher degree research supervisors. These reflective groups draw upon the breadth of experience and resources of group members and, as a facilitator, there is a definite reward when 'your' group has developed to the point it no longer needs your involvement as the group is functioning effectively.

Group working challenges tradition and hierarchy

Group working for supervision, reflection and developing the individual's abilities, skills and knowledge mirrors other shifts in thinking. Traditionally, supervision and supervisory practices have been viewed from a somewhat essentialist perspective, such as that described by Maggs and Biley (2000, p.192) who propose that supervision can 'develop competence in practice, protect the patient/client and provide structured support for the professional'.

More recently, authors have questioned an approach to supervision that is inherently hierarchical and process oriented (Shanley and Stevenson 2006). Stevenson (2005, pp.525–526) highlights that:

> '. . . modernist, hierarchical supervision has a stranglehold on CS (clinical supervision) practice, yet, it can hardly be said to be unproblematic; it is heavily critiqued from both outside and within the post-modern turn'.

She proposes a post-modern, social constructionist approach to clinical supervision which challenges the traditional functional normative–formative–restorative approach to clinical supervision, since this traditional approach 'implies a linear progress towards the practically perfect practitioner' (Stevenson 2005, p.520). She proposes that 'egalitarian consultation meetings' (ECMs) promote a non-hierarchical, dialogic approach (Stevenson 2005, p.520) which acknowledge the 'practitioner as expert on the person in context' (p.526) and where 'radical talk (can) occur in relation to how practice might be better organised' (p.527). The notion of the practitioner having expertise on the person-in-context is important. The practitioner who has close clinical contact with the patient (the person-in-context) is (arguably) better positioned than a more distant supervisor, to bring with his/her clinically grounded insights, understandings and situated knowledge of the patient to reflective meetings. The

ECM approach that Stevenson advocates in relation to clinical supervision has huge resonance for all types of reflective groups.

Group working: an overview of the good, the bad and the ugly

Group working has many advantages, but before embarking on group reflection it is important to appreciate that it brings with it not only benefits, such as a more democratic approach to reflection, but also challenges and some difficulties. Some of these are summarised in Box 6.1.

Box 6.1   Overview of the good, the bad and the ugly of reflective group work

- Group work can encourage a democratic sharing of ideas.
- Group reflection can encourage more ideas to develop and flourish.
- Using imagination and creativity in reflective groups can open up new ways of thinking and suggest new solutions.
- Group work makes reflection a more public activity than one-to-one reflection.
- One aspect of the facilitator's role is to ensure that group members feel safe.
- Group work may result in participants selecting safe topics and not discussing the more difficult issues.
- Group reflection can offer benefits to nurses at all stages of their careers.
- Group reflection can promote a sense of professional identity.
- Group reflection may cause anticipatory anxiety.
- The aims of the group should be explicit and negotiated.
- Group work can be uncomfortable at times.
- A supportive group environment requires active effort from the participants and facilitator.
- Group time needs to be protected and groups should start and end on time.
- Confidentiality and anonymity need to be considered especially when practice is discussed.
- Good facilitators should be working towards making themselves redundant within 'their' group.
- Facilitation is a skilled role and facilitators need support.
- Group work may result in participants experiencing vicarious distress.

Beyond the status quo

Whilst one-to-one approaches can be a powerful means of providing individual attention and focus, there is also the potential for supervisees to feel isolated and reliant on the competence of their supervisors (Platzer 2004). One-to-one approaches used without due care and consideration of feelings can become one-*on*-one sessions. Group work can be helpful as individuals within a group can offer different experiences and ideas and 'many heads are better than one' (Winship and Hardy 1999, p.312). Group work offers an approach that can complement or potentially replace individual, one-to-one approaches to promoting reflection and providing supervision. Clouder and Sellars (2004, p.266) note that clinical supervision has the 'potential to move beyond preserving the status quo to enhancing practice' and they also note that its 'full potential . . . *might* be recognised more readily in a group supervision context' (emphasis added).

Effective group working aims to ensure a more democratic approach in which multiple *ways of knowing* as well as multiple *sources of knowing* are acknowledged and drawn upon. Peer support, peer feedback and a democratic sharing of experience can be nurtured within a group (Rolfe *et al.* 2001).

Creativity and imagination in groups

Effective group working can also open up other avenues – such as the use of imagination within reflective practice groups – to support change. Williams and Walker (2003, p.134) report on how imagination can open up the 'possible options of behaving in future similar situations' and 'the possible outcomes if these different options were to be completed'. A core aspect of using imagination in a reflective group is using the group as a means of grounding imagined possibilities by discussing these and establishing their suitability.

An example from a group setting focused on the challenges that Phoebe, a newly qualified nurse working in a high-dependency unit, was experiencing. She had described to the group how vulnerable she felt when the patients' relatives were watching her when she was providing nursing care. She explained that she felt quite confident most of the time but that her confidence drained away when the relatives arrived. The group offered their own experiences and most reported that they had experienced similar feelings of exposure and anxiety when they had been newly qualified and then shared stories about how they had coped. One of the group members – Tilly – explained that she had managed her own nerves by pretending she was a sunflower. This slightly bizarre response caused a lot of giggling and this in itself helped put Phoebe even more at ease. Tilly explained that during her first summer as a staff nurse she had felt much the same as Phoebe and had had worried a lot about whether or not she was ever going to be able to be really confident. She described walking home through the park one evening and seeing some pansies that had been flattened by some children playing football. She said that, 'At that moment in time, I knew exactly how those pansies felt – squashed!' Tilly went on to say, 'But the thing was, in the same bed there were a whole lot of other flowers that weren't squashed and the best of the lot were the sunflowers. They were gorgeous – tall and bonny looking and just being themselves'. The following day at work she started to feel worried and anxious, but the image of the sunflowers and the pansies came into her mind. Without thinking too much about it at the time she said she decided to be like a sunflower; stand tall and face things. She described how the image really helped, it made her feel more positive, actually stand taller and feel more confident. The group were able to see the sense of 'pretending to be a sunflower' and this sparked a lively discussion of whether this would work for other people and what flowers they would choose. Phoebe thought having something to visualise would be helpful as she felt she 'just got too focused on feeling like the relatives were watching her'. Reflecting within the group helped Phoebe think about what she was worried about and also helped to give her a visual strategy for getting through a difficult time. At the next group meeting, Phoebe pulled a postcard from her pocket of a really cheerful orange gerbera daisy. She had found Tilly's idea really useful. She explained it had felt a bit odd to begin with to visualise the daisy when she got stressed, but the daisy was such a strong and cheerful image it had helped a lot. She had started to feel different about being watched and was starting to develop her confidence.

Groups: simply cheaper, not better?

Whilst imagination and creativity can occur in one-to-one situations, there is a greater potential for these to flourish in group settings, where encouragement from other members of the group can help open up a creative streak that had previously been untapped. However, whilst group reflection/supervision has many strengths and the potential to reflect in different ways, it is not a panacea to any or all the ills associated with one-to-one approaches. Groups can be good, but equally they can be bad/ugly if they are ineffectively supported. White and Winstanley's (2006) study examined the cost and resource implications of one-to-one and group clinical supervision. Slight differences (in favour of one-to-one) were found in relation to the importance/value of clinical supervision and the scores on the Manchester Clinical Supervision (CS) subscale, although these were not clinically significant. However, they did note that cost savings could occur with groups as they would take less time to run and, overall, would need fewer supervisors.

Power, groups and facilitation

An important difference between individual and group approaches is that group work takes reflection and supervision out of a relatively private domain (between the two people involved) and opens it up into a much more public domain (between group members). Used badly it can compound problems of powerlessness and can expose participants in a way that one-to-one supervision is less likely to. The 'contract' moves from being between two people to being between all members of the group. Everyone has to 'act well' for group work to be really effective. Reflecting on our personal experience of working with groups, facilitators need to be vigilant for problems that may arise within the group. Group work is most effective when the conditions are right. A crucial condition is the involvement of a skilled facilitator whose role is to prepare participants, create a supportive environment and encourage engagement with the process.

Up until recently, the role of facilitator has most often been adopted by a senior person either based within the practice setting or from an associated education setting. The drawback of this somewhat hierarchical-external-expert approach is that the reflection and/or supervision activity may become muddled with line management and 'innocent questions asked by the supervisor (e.g., "How is the case going?") can be interpreted as surveillance' and seen to be 'coercive' (Stevenson 2005, p.522–523). Group participants exposed to such perceived risks will inevitably 'select, interpret and sanitise issues brought to clinical supervision' (Clouder and Sellars 2004, p.266). Whilst this holding back of issues could be seen as a mechanism employed by participants who perceive themselves as being less powerful and/or expert than the facilitator (or other group participants), it can in reality be a very effective, albeit subtle, means of exerting passive power over the group. Passive or active misuse/abuse of power is detrimental to group dynamics. Some groups overcome potential power issues by making membership relatively homogenous (similar grades or experiences); other groups see the potential richness in a diversity of experience and knowledge that a more heterogeneous group can hold. More diverse groups may generate and share greater insights into organisational culture and practice that give rise to more opportunities for genuine learning that could positively impact on practice.

Group dynamics can be affected by power issues. Much of the work associated with group reflection and supervision, specifically within nursing, is linked to action learning and the use of action learning sets/groups. In this sense it is sometimes difficult to separate the benefits of the group work per se from the other activities that the participants may be engaged in.

Benefits of group work

In terms of the good, the bad and the ugly of group work, a number of good things or benefits are evident in the literature. These benefits range from developing capacity and confidence, being supportive, helping to illuminate and enhance aspects of practice and improving the patient's/

client's experience of care. These advantages have potential for nurses at varying stages within their careers; from students taking their first steps towards developing an understanding of their professional role (Gould and Masters 2004) to experienced practitioners taking on the challenges of driving nursing practice forward through their leadership skills (Alleyne and Jumaa 2007).

With a focus on trained staff working within an intensive care unit, Lindahl and Norberg (2002, p.816) note that group supervision was 'helpful and supportive in managing professional and personally demanding complex nursing care'. The participants valued the cohesiveness that developed as a result of working within the group which they felt could not have been developed had supervision been managed on a one-to-one basis. The participants experienced 'improved self image' and were able to share their 'relationships with patients and patients' next of kin' (Lindahl and Norberg 2002, p.816). Saarikoski et al. (2006, p.283) found that group supervision/reflection compared to one-to-one provided support to mental health nursing students who became less anxious about their ability to manage the 'unfamiliar emotional and psychological demands of practice'. In this same study they also noted that group supervision was more positive in fostering a sense of professional identity than the one-to-one control group (Saarikoski et al. 2006). Certainly, our own experience supports the value of group-based reflection for promoting a sense of professional identity.

Holm et al. (1998, p.109) found that process-oriented group supervision sessions which aimed to help develop nursing identity in nursing students had a number of beneficial effects, including 'sharing experiences of actions and reactions' and the students also 'learnt to listen more actively to each other and to achieve greater integration of their own and others' experiences of work'. Group supervision in Arvidsson et al.'s study (2000, p.184–185) focused on supporting psychiatric nurses to develop competence as professionals. The findings show that the 'nurses gained increased trust in their own abilities, feelings and work performance. They became more courageous, dared more and worked independently to a greater extent...' and that over time, supervision 'strengthened the psychiatric nurses' trust in themselves and their professional competence...(and reflecting)...upon the relation between theory and practice provided the nurses with opportunities to increase their professional competence'.

Anticipatory anxiety and challenges to group reflection

Whilst participants in group supervision will generally report positive aspects, group settings may cause anticipatory anxiety. This anxiety can be seen as one of the 'bad/ugly' aspects of group work since if it is not managed effectively it can stop a group from working well. Some anxiety is natural and to be expected and may reflect previous negative experiences of supervision (Walsh *et al.* 2003); good facilitation can do a great deal to overcome this in the initial meetings. Alleyne and Jumaa (2007, p.235) reflect on the way that their participants demonstrated evidence of strategic thinking and action after 'effective socialisation and acceptance of the GCS (group clinical supervision) sessions' in which they were involved for their management development. It would seem that some careful preparation was used to facilitate these participants' first steps into group-based clinical supervision. Within this study 'executive co-coaching' was a crucial element of preparation; this involved 'building an alliance between the coach and the client using stakeholder analysis and management' (p.234).

Although facilitators and other stakeholders may see the positive aspects of group working, these do not necessarily always appear to be obvious to potential participants. However, this shift from anxiety to acceptance is evident in many of the published studies and our own experiences broadly mirror these. Lindgren *et al.* (2005), for example, note in their study of group supervision of Swedish student nurses that 25% had negative expectations about group supervision before they commenced it. At the end of their group supervision programme all of the students felt that group supervision had been an 'important support to them during their training and almost everyone wanted to participate in group supervision in the future, when they had become registered nurses' (Lindgren *et al.* 2005, p.827). Jones (2003, 2006) also notes that within his study focusing on hospice nurses' experiences of group supervision that some nurses were reticent about the prospect of discussing difficult and sensitive aspects of their practice. He states that the participants 'found aspects of group work anxiety invoking and took time to trust and settle into the group task because of personal concerns . . . (and that) initial interactions suggested that psychological and social defences were preventing group members from sharing experiences openly' (Jones 2006, p.161). Similar findings were identified by Platzer *et al.* (2000, p.1005) who noted issues relating to vulnerability with some of the post-registration students who were trying to develop reflective practice and who 'took a long time to develop a sense of trust whereby students felt able to explore their practice without feeling that they should have always done things according to the book'.

From our own practice of working with groups we have found that an initial characteristic of most groups is reticence. This is often evident regardless of whether we are working with first-year pre-registration students or with doctoral students. Indeed our experience suggests that groups composed of senior and expert nurses can create specific challenges to the facilitators as the participants may feel they have more to lose and feel more vulnerable about revealing aspects of themselves to other participants. As one participant explained during an early reflective group meeting for senior nurses:

'It's hard enough just to be sat here, let alone contemplating "spill-ing all" to people you don't know well. I spend most of my days in work, trying to be a role model, leading by example and yet in this room I'm expected to peel back some of my defences and talk reflectively about my practice. That feels almost impossibly hard at the moment. I can see the point of it. I like the sound of it. But I'm not sure I'm ready for it'.

Perhaps unsurprisingly, this opened a floodgate; other participants showed their support and many of them confirmed that they were also feeling hesitant and anxious about sharing their experiences and feelings. They equally assured her that they also thought that even if it felt 'impos-sibly hard' it would be worth the effort. One of the other participants summed this up by saying,

'Practice is often so demanding and draining and yet there's not many people you can turn to for support, people who you can trust. I don't feel I can talk to the people I manage about feeling angry about some things – that wouldn't be professional. And I certainly don't feel like I could talk to my line manager! So if things work out, this group could be absolutely brilliant for me – potentially a life and sanity saver'.

This group did indeed blossom into a supportive structure; where par-ticipants shared difficulties they were facing, provided different perspec-tives and solutions, provided support for each other and reduced the feelings of isolation experienced in senior management.

Explaining the purpose of a reflective group

Ensuring that every member of a group (from the very enthusiastic to the more cynical and resistant) has a clear idea of the purpose of the group is absolutely crucial. Both the group's aims and the aims of the individuals should be negotiated and made explicit. Whilst the facilitator will have a key role in ensuring that this happens, the participants themselves have a responsibility to each other right from the start. Perhaps unsurprisingly, Eraut (2004, p.49) notes that 'members of a group have very different agendas' even when the purpose seems clear within specific reflective episodes. Our own experience would support this as we have often found that participants may bring an issue to a group that is particularly current and pertinent to them. Whilst it might be valuable to pursue an issue such as a proposed ward closure, it needs to be done in a way that has relevance to everyone in the group. If this is not possible, we have found that the best thing is to provide a short amount of time for the issue to be acknowledged by the group before moving on to the actual focus of the group. One way of dealing with this is to provide participants with a 'two minute steam' which gives them the chance to get something out of their system before starting the actual reflective session.

Membership issues

Some groups have a fixed or closed membership whilst others may adopt a more fluid approach. Neither is the perfect approach and the choice ultimately is dependent on the reason(s) for the group forming, contextual factors, the degree of sensitivity of the issues to be discussed and, at a more pragmatic level, the practicalities involved. Whilst trust may develop more easily in a closed group this should not be the primary reason for closed membership. Open groups, which necessarily have to be more flexible and accommodating, may more genuinely reflect everyday practice as the 'rivalries and micro politics of the workplace cannot easily be put aside' (Eraut 2004, p.49). Winship and Hardy (1999) note that some of the conflicts and difficulties that occur in group work can prepare nurses for dealing with the sorts of conflicts that occur in clinical practice situations. They further wryly note that even for the 'most inveterate of optimistic staff, there were times when the group was inescapably excruciating and difficult to bear as conflicts surfaced and harsh words were shared' (Winship and Hardy 1999, p.309). Groups where people are already known to each other, for example, when they are made up of staff working in a particular team or setting may benefit from that existing knowledge of each other. However, a limitation of this is that 'colleagues may hold similar views, restricting the extent to which any benefits of supervision are experienced by the team as whole' (Cleary and Freeman 2005, p.491).

The challenge and rewards of group reflection

It is clear that reflective groups are a challenge and not an easy option, but the rewards can be commensurately large. Challenge is intrinsic to reflection; without exploring the conflict and contradictions that arise then reflection is limited and participants do not move beyond habitual responses (McGill and Beaty 2001). Interestingly, Walsh *et al.* (2003, p.39) note that community nurses in the group they were studying believed that in their 'effort to be supportive they did not sufficiently challenge each other. This in turn meant that their ability to reflect upon and critique practice was compromised'. They reported that this group intended to develop the level of challenge in the future without damaging the supportive environment. Developing a supportive environment does not just happen; it requires active effort from all of the participants, it builds over time and some risks have to be taken. Each group will create and sustain their own supportive environment as it is dependent on the experiences, expectations and commitments of the individuals within the group. As a group develops a sense of safety, then the boundaries can be pushed and in our own experience this is the point at which reflection can really start to fly.

The challenges of group work include ensuring that every participant is engaged within the group. This is often linked with ensuring that an appropriate amount of time is available so that reflection can occur in sufficient depth and that the stories and/or issues that are shared are addressed appropriately. Ensuring that no one person monopolises the group is an important part of facilitation. Lindahl and Norberg (2002, p.816) identified that time constraints with the groups they were research-ing hindered 'deep narratives'. Group size and time constraints mean that every group has to work within limits on the length and detail of the narratives that can be shared. Whilst in a large group every participant might be able to say something, short superficial presentations constrain the quality and depth of any reflection (Eraut 2004). Whilst there are no hard and fast rules about group size it is important to consider the effects that group size has on group dynamics and the ability to reflect in depth. Groups with around eight members have a good chance of functioning well; relationships can be developed and sharing of deep narratives can occur and participants do not feel too fazed by contributing within a group of this size.

Running a group: ground rules and other pragmatic issues

Running a reflective group is challenging and there is no recipe for getting it right. However, there are a number of areas that anyone who is thinking of facilitating a group should consider (see Box 6.2 for an overview of core principles for facilitating group reflection).

Group time and commitment to the group

Pragmatically the facilitator, in liaison with the group members, needs to determine how often the group needs to meet to keep the momentum going. Saarikoski et al. (2006) notes that her group of student nurses was less than cohesive, which she proposes resulted from them only meeting five times as a group during the course of a 5-week clinical placement. The group also has to determine what level of priority the group activity is accorded, so that the time and space for the group is protected from other concerns. Protecting group time is important (Platzer 2004) as this is an essential prerequisite to ensuring that the group actually does happen and that people within the group have an equitable opportunity to contribute. Commitment to the group is usually one of the ground rules that the group will set and aim to abide by. Other ground rules

Box 6.2   Principles for facilitating group reflection.
(Developed and adapted from 'Behaviours which will facilitate
learning', Mumford 1996, p.8)

- Ensuring everyone in the group has a fair and appropriate share of the available time.
- Being non-defensive about own actions and reflections.
- Supporting the issues/concerns that group members raise.
- Being open in initiating and responding to issues.
- Being analytical and thoughtful about the reflections raised.
- Adopting a challenging but constructive approach to eliciting further information.
- Listening effectively.
- Summarising accurately without undue interpretation.
- Being creative, imaginative and solution oriented in response to identified challenges/problems.
- Being insightful about the reflections that are being shared.
- Being able to take risks and being aware that you are taking them and are aware of potential consequences.
- Using strengths/resourcefulness of group members and not overrelying on own experiences/expertise.
- Motivating and encouraging all members of the group and valuing individuals' contributions.
- Supporting less vocal, less confident members of the group to share their experiences.
- Praising people's efforts.
- Providing direction as appropriate.
- Developing ground rules with the group that are meaningful and contextualised and sustainable.
- Knowing when to keep quiet – valuing silence.

Chapter 6

usually focus on issues of confidentiality, respecting other people's opinions, not interrupting, and preparing appropriately for the group. These rules are relatively easy to write and can be equally easy to commit to, but it is often more difficult to consistently put them into practice. The dynamic nature of group discussion means that adhering to ground rules is anything but effortless; this in itself can be a good source of learning and reflection. Issues relating to patient care, therapeutic interventions and professional accountability may be pertinent topics to reflect upon, but they can give rise to particular tensions and implications. Table 6.1 provides an overview of the key processes/phases in facilitating a reflective group.

Table 6.1 Overview of key processes/phases in facilitating a reflective group

Before the meeting	• The facilitator needs to find a comfortable venue that is conducive to reflective discussion. • Invite participants to the group. • Provide participants with appropriate information about the aims of the group.
At the start of the first meeting	• Create a safe and positive environment for the participants in the group in which they can work and share their ideas. • Use 'ice breakers' with the participants to help them get to know each other. This is also useful in a group where people know each other. These ice breaker activities need not be complicated but can involve asking questions about each others' areas of practice or something nothing to do with professional life such as where they went on their last holiday. Sharing this information with the group starts to provide some insight into their practice as well as revealing something about the participants as individuals. Taking notes can help act as an effective aide memoire. • Ensure that participants have an underpinning knowledge of the reflective process and how it will work within a group setting.
Develop the ground rules	• Every group will develop their own ground rules based on what is important to them. However, some rules are fairly fundamental and seen in most reflective practice groups; these include confidentiality, listening, being non-judgmental, having the right to stay silent, and starting and ending the group on time.
Group discussion time	• Enable participants to contribute and recall events they wish to discuss. Ensure participants appreciate that they can share incidents of good practice as well as situations where they feel they did not do as well as they wanted to. • Analyse the issues using your chosen reflective model/framework. • Explore the theory–practice links. • Identify the lessons to learn from the incidents discussed. • Identify actions that can be taken to enhance practice.
At the end of the meeting	• Summarise the group activity. • Identify any actions that participants need to take in preparation for the next meeting and/or as a result of this meeting. • Thank everyone for their attendance. • Check that all the participants are okay, particularly if anyone appeared distressed, angry or very withdrawn, for example.

Confidentiality

The assurance of confidentiality has to be balanced against a nurse's duty of care and adherence to the professional Code of Conduct (Nursing and Midwifery Council 2004). However, in these circumstances if it is likely that confidentiality will need to be breached, then this should normally need to be discussed within the group. Listening effectively to other group members is essential and is particularly important when one participant may be recalling a complex critical practice incident. Unless the group members listen carefully, they will be less able to contribute thoughtfully to the reflective discussion arising from the shared incident. Recalling and sharing an incident lays the person who is relating the incident open to the scrutiny and judgement of others. Apart from rare incidents where it is clear that someone was acting unprofessionally, it is important that participants respect the decisions made by other people and understand that the actions they took occurred in a particular setting and context. This does not mean to say that the actions taken and responses to these actions cannot be reflected upon and practice improved in some way.

One core ground rule that does not always appear in text books is the imperative to start and end the group on time. Busy practitioners often state that 'lack of time' is a key reason for not wanting to participate in group reflection. Therefore it is really important for the facilitator to start and finish the group on time. This may mean the facilitator having to satisfactorily bring a lively discussion to an end so that the meeting can finish on time. This can be done by documenting ongoing issues and assuring participants that they will be picked up at the next meeting or, where appropriate, arranging to meet up with individuals to discuss them between the scheduled group meetings.

Facilitation and 'flying solo'

Although many groups will draw upon the skills of a facilitator in their early stages, most facilitators should be working towards making themselves redundant within the group. Otherwise there is a possibility that a paradox might be created within a group that is reflecting on issues such as empowerment, independence and autonomy whilst remaining dependent on facilitation. This approach is particularly true for action learning sets where part of the facilitator's role is to model effective styles and approaches to questions and communication (McGill and Beaty 2001). Interestingly in Stark's (2006) study of using action learning for professional development she comments on clear disparities in relation to her groups being able to 'fly solo'. She notes that the 'educators' regular attendance at set meetings enabled them to quickly learn effective group processes and complete the facilitation transference to themselves as a group. Whereas the more erratic attendance at the nurses'

set meetings . . . resulted in these sets needing more sustained facilitation to keep the projects moving forward' (Stark 2006, p.27).

Facilitators need the chance to reflect too

Rolfe *et al.* (2001) note that facilitators need supervision for themselves.
Facilitating a group is not an easy role and it demands an ethical and
moral response from the facilitator. Agelii *et al.* (2000, p.358) in their
study of the ethical dimensions of group supervision conclude that one
of the responsibilities of the supervisor/facilitator is 'to create a moral
reflective mental space'. It requires skill to help participants make their
own decisions and conclusions concerning incidents from practice. Given
that the incidents chosen for discussion may be distressing, facilitators
may find themselves, as we have done on occasion, on an emotional
rollercoaster confronting many difficult scenarios. Interestingly, whilst
supervision is seen as being an important tool in dealing with the vicarious distress and trauma that can be encountered in practice (Sexton
1999; Bell *et al.* 2003), there is much less written about how facilitators
should deal with their own vicarious distress that may arise as a result of
listening to a series of traumatic incidents. Even less acknowledgement
has been made about possible vicarious group distress and how to deal
with it. At the very least facilitators need to be aware of the potential of
being overwhelmed by difficult stories and take care that they have
access to support for their own emotional and professional needs.

Reflective group work in action

Joan's story

Having gained an overview of the processes involved in facilitating a
group, Joan's story of 'rescuing a patient' on her way to work (see Box
6.3) is presented as a way of sharing the type of incident that may be
discussed during a group meeting. This example is shared with the permission of Joan and the other group members. Pseudonyms have been
used and client details have been changed to ensure anonymity.

  Joan's story and her reflections occurred within a group she had been
reflecting with for a few weeks and she felt safe to disclose not only the
incident but also her feelings, as she felt confident that the group would
be non-judgmental even if they disagreed with her actions.

Areas for reflection and how Joan and Michael felt

After telling her story, Joan identified a number of interlinked areas that
she wanted to reflect on with her colleagues in the group. She felt there
were issues of vulnerability and safety to discuss as well as issues of
accountability and autonomy.

Box 6.3   Joan's story

Joan, a staff nurse on a rehabilitation unit, often cycled to work. One evening, even though a little concerned about being late for work, she noticed a man sitting in a wheelchair outside a pub. Although, the man had his hat pulled down over his face Joan recognised him as Michael, a patient from her own unit. Not being sure of why she felt a little apprehensive, Joan got off her bicycle and went over to speak to Michael. As soon as she got close to him, she realised something was wrong. Even though it was a summer evening, Michael was very cold and he could hardly speak. He gradually explained that he'd had an argument with the friend who had had taken him out for a drink and that his friend had left him outside the pub 'hours ago'. Without his friend's help, Michael, who was tetraplegic, had no way of getting himself back to the unit. Based on her clinical experience Joan realised that Michael wasn't simply cold but becoming hypothermic; she could see his condition deteriorating. Joan knew she needed to act quickly and so she rang for an ambulance.

As she waited for the ambulance and reassured Michael and tried to keep him warm, she was worried about being late for her shift but felt she couldn't just leave Michael as he was already distressed. She followed the ambulance to the hospital. Michael was moved from his usual bed space to a high observation area on the unit and wrapped in a space blanket. Joan continued to care for him during the night, performing his observations, reassuring him that he was getting better and listening to Michael's concerns. She was relieved to see during the course of the night that his condition improved and temperature returned to normal. Michael told Joan that he knew he was really lucky that she'd seen him and stopped and called for an ambulance.

Vulnerability and safety

Joan talked about how vulnerable Michael had seemed to be and how surprised she had been to find him 'abandoned and alone'. As she, Joan, was relating this story to the group she became upset as she realised that if she had not seen Michael and acted the way she did the consequences could have been serious for him. She was also surprised by the way his friend had acted. By leaving Michael on his own, his friend had unknowingly set off a chain of events that could have resulted in very different consequences for Michael. The situation in some ways seemed worse since Michael usually managed the challenges of his disability well and ensured that he was safe. Joan also described that although she 'knew what she had to do and recognised that Michael was becoming hypothermic, that she felt vulnerable as she was assessing Michael and making decisions outside of her usual clinical environment'.

Chapter 6

Accountability and autonomy

Joan wanted to reflect on her feelings of worry about whether or not the unit protocol for ensuring that patients who were away from the ward was safe. The protocol aimed to ensure that patients only left the unit in the care of people who would act in a responsible way. It seemed to Joan that Michael's friend had not been aware of how vulnerable Michael was to getting cold and how he was dependent on him. Joan was clear that Michael (and his friend) would need help and support to avoid a similar situation occurring in the future. Joan also expressed concern that the protocol had let Michael down in some way. She saw issues relating to the unit's responsibility to prevent Michael leaving the ward and to her accountability for her intervention; she also wondered if Michael should be considered to be responsible for his own actions to any extent.

As an experienced staff nurse she fully appreciated the balance between being over-protective of patients and giving patients, like Michael, the opportunity to maintain social networks and enjoy social outings with friends.

Overwhelmingly, Joan was relieved that she had noticed Michael and, by calling for an ambulance, had ensured that she had got him back into a safe environment. Joan reflected on the fact that although it had felt strange making decisions 'on the pavement', she had felt confident that her assessment of Michael's condition was based on her long experience with patients with this type of disability.

Other group members' responses

When Joan became distressed most of the group were supportive of her actions and expressed empathy and praise for the way she had handled the situation. Some members of the group appeared to be reticent about the situation and did not initially join actively in the discussions. However, one group member felt that since Joan was off duty when she found Michael a more appropriate course of action would have been to have rung for an ambulance but to have carried on to work, asking someone at the scene to stay with Michael. This different view challenged both Joan and the group. The facilitator encouraged group members to consider the potential benefits had Joan not stayed with Michael, considering that, since the incident made Joan late for work, a valuable member of the night shift was missing. Joan reflected on this carefully. She decided that the actions she had taken were the right ones and that she had acted in Michael's best interest, especially since he was deteriorating. She felt that the successful and safe outcome was based on the actions that she had taken. Although most of the group had been supportive of what she had done, Joan and the rest of the group appreciated that they had learnt a lot from the challenging comment.

The group encouraged Joan to tell her story and helped Joan to think through the issues even though it was clear that it was painful at times. It brought the group members face-to-face with the consequences of deciding when patients were sufficiently prepared for outings and they thought through the ways in which they could develop even better practice in preparing friends and family to accompany patients.

Reflecting on how Michael felt

Joan also reflected on Michael's feelings and how he had responded to the situation. Michael described feeling shocked at what had happened and upset that his friend had just gone off and left him after the argument. He had always trusted his friend who had taken him out to the pub on other occasions. Initially he was angry with his friend, but he was glad to find out that his friend had come back to the pub to make sure he was okay even though by the time he had arrived, Michael had been taken to hospital by ambulance. Michael was very thankful that Joan had found him and acted as she had. He was aware that he had inadvertently put himself in a dangerous situation and that he needed to be more careful in the future. Michael felt that the episode had reinforced what he already knew, that as a disabled man with poor temperature control, he must take care of himself and be sure that people around him are fully aware of the risks.

Learning from reflections on the incident

Everyone in the group learned something from the incident. Joan was glad that she had interrupted her journey to work. She had acted quickly in a crisis situation, she had used her clinical skills of observation and assessment outside of the hospital setting and she had ensured that Michael was returned to a safe environment. Joan learned that she could act quickly and cope in a crisis situation. Joan also discovered that her colleagues thought she had acted well and that they would have felt similarly concerned.

One of the early discussions led by the facilitator had addressed issues of managing distress within the group and how, when stories or incidents are told, they often evoke different perspectives from people who might disagree with the actions that had been taken. As a member of the group, Joan had, to a degree, been forewarned about how she might feel confused and unsettled by being challenged and so these feelings were not too problematic to deal with.

Other people in the group learned about how they felt they might respond in a similar situation and also about the consequences that can occur if a patient and his or her friend are not appropriately prepared for an outing away from the unit. The protocol became more of a live document than a piece of paper. The group also learned that not everyone would have acted in the same way and that a different course of action might not necessarily have been wrong.

Summary

Joan's story might not seem very complex. She saw a patient who needed help and she responded by calling for an ambulance. Joan did not do anything particularly heroic. However, the incident that Joan described showed how exposed she felt about intervening in public, and how many competing concerns and worries can result from the seemingly simple action of stopping to help someone on your way to work. What was interesting from this group reflection was the way in which other people responded and the perspectives they offered. Interestingly over the course of subsequent group meetings, elements of Joan's story continued to be reflected on or referred back to in other people's reflections.

Some critics might think that Joan could have come to the same conclusions simply by reflecting on the incident on her own or by taking it to a one-to-one supervision session. Perhaps this is true, but it is unlikely that either of these other two approaches would have resulted in the breadth of support that she gained or the variety and nuances of experiences shared. Neither of the other approaches would have resulted in the breadth of learning that occurred. A substantive advantage of group reflection is that not only does the individual sharing the initial incident explore, consider and learn but also so do all the other members of the group.

Conclusion – many hands . . . or too many cooks?

Within this chapter we have explored the nature of group reflection, supervision and learning as well as the key ways in which group reflection may be different to the reflection that occurs in one-to-one situations. Since groups are likely to be 'here to stay' it is important to acknowledge the potential benefits that accrue from the dynamics and relationships that develop between members of a group. However, it is also important to note that group reflection is complex, challenging and potentially more democratic than one-to-one approaches. The adage that 'many hands make light work' could be true within group reflection and supervision; the range of perspectives that can be shared can illuminate problems and provide a breadth and depth of resource that is difficult to match in a one-to-one setting. However, another adage comes to mind – 'too many cooks spoil the broth'. Ineffective group work can arise from a number of factors including poorly managed contributions from participants, active and passive resistance to the group and lack of focus.

Group work is powerful and fragile. It has enormous potential; it requires commitment and courage from the participants and the ability to create a safe and secure environment from the facilitator. As group supervision starts to become more embedded within day-to-day practice we believe its potential will start to be realised and the rewards will be reaped.

References

Abma, T.A. (2007) Situated learning in communities of practice: evaluation of coercion in psychiatry as a case. *Evaluation*, **13**, 32–47.

Agelii, E. Kennergren, B., Severinsson, E. and Berthold, H. (2000) Ethical dimensions of supervision: the supervisor's experiences. *Nursing Ethics*, **7**, 350–359.

Alleyne, J.O. and Jumaa, M.O. (2007) Building the capacity for evidence-based clinical nursing leadership: the role of executive co-coaching and group clinical supervision for quality patient services. *Journal of Nursing Management*, **15**, 230–243.

Armstrong, A. and Foley, P. (2003) Foundations for a learning organization: organization learning mechanisms. *The Learning Organization: An International Journal*, **10**, 74–82.

Arvidsson, B., Lofgren, H. and Fridlund, B. (2000) Psychiatric nurses' conceptions of how group supervision in nursing care influences their professional competence. *Journal of Nursing Management*, **8**, 175–185.

Bell, H., Kulkarni, S. and Dalton, L. (2003) Organizational prevention of vicarious trauma. *Families in Society: The Journal of Contemporary Human Services*, **84**, 463–470.

Booth, A., Sutton, A. and Falzon, L. (2003) Working together: supporting projects through action learning. *Health Information and Libraries Journal*, **20**, 225–231.

Brennan, J. and Little, B. (2007) Liberation by degrees. *The Times Higher Education Supplement*, 11 May, 6–7.

Brown, B.A., Harte, J. and Warnes, A.-M. (2007) Developing the health care workforce: a comparison of two work-based learning models. *Education + Training*, **49**, 193–200.

Burton, J. (2004) *Understanding and Promoting Work Based Learning in Primary Care*, 2nd edn. Radcliffe Medical Press, Oxford, pp. 199–201.

Cleary, M. and Freeman, A. (2005) The cultural realities of clinical supervision in an acute inpatient mental health setting. *Issues in Mental Health Nursing*, **26**, 489–505.

Clouder, L. and Sellars, J. (2004) Reflective practice and clinical supervision: an interprofessional perspective. *Journal of Advanced Nursing*, **46**, 262–269.

Court, D. (2003) Quest for patient safety in a challenging environment. *The Australian and New Zealand Journal of Obstetrics and Gynaecology*, **43**, 97–100.

Cunningham, G. and Kitson, A. (2000) An evaluation of the RCN Clinical Leadership Development Programme: part 1. *Nursing Standard*, **15**, 34–37.

Dealey, C., Moss, H., Marshall, J. and Elcoat, C. (2007) Auditing the impact of implementing the Modern Matron role in an acute teaching trust. *Journal of Nursing Management*, **15**, 22–33.

Dewar, B.J. and Walker, E. (1999) Experiential learning: issues for supervision. *Journal of Advanced Nursing*, **30**, 1459–1467.

Douglas, S. and Machin, T. (2004) A model for setting up interdisciplinary collaborative working in groups: lessons from an experience of action learning. *Journal of Psychiatric and Mental Health Nursing*, **11**, 189–193.

Eraut, M. (2004) The practice of reflection. *Learning in Health and Social Care*, **3**, 47–52.

Flanagan, J., Baldwin, S. and Clarke, D. (2000) Work-based learning as a means of developing and assessing nursing competence. *Journal of Clinical Nursing*, **9**, 360–368.

Garbett, R., Hardy, S. Manley, K., Titchen, A. and McCormack, B. (2007) Developing a qualitative approach to 360-degree feedback to aid understanding and development of clinical expertise. *Journal of Nursing Management*, **15**, 342–347.

Gherardi, S. (2001) From organizational learning to practice-based knowing. *Human Relations*, **54**, 131–139.

Gould, B. and Masters, H. (2004) Learning to make sense: the use of critical incident analysis in facilitated reflective groups of mental health student nurses. *Learning in Health and Social Care*, **3**, 53–63.

Hardacre, J.E. and Keep, J. (2003) From intent to impact: developing clinical leaders for service improvement. *Learning in Health and Social Care*, **2**, 169–176.

Hardy, S., Titchen, A. and Manley, K. (2007) Patient narratives in the investigation and development of nursing practice expertise: a potential for transformation. *Nursing Inquiry*, **14**, 80–88.

Heiskanen, T. (2007) A knowledge-building community for public sector professionals. *The Journal of Workplace Learning*, **16**, 370–384.

Holm, A., Lantz, I. and Severinsson, E. (1998) Nursing students' experiences of the effects of continual process-oriented group supervision. *Journal of Nursing Management*, **6**, 105–113.

Jones, A. (2003) Some benefits experienced by hospice nurses from group clinical supervision. *European Journal of Cancer Care*, **12**, 224–232.

Jones, A. (2006) Group-format clinical supervision for hospice nurses. *European Journal of Cancer Care*, **15**, 155–162.

Kelly, T.B., Lowndes, A. and Tolson, D. (2005) Advancing stages of group development: the case of a virtual nursing community of practice groups. *Group Work: An Interdisciplinary Journal for Working with Groups*, **15**, 17–38.

Lathlean, J. and Le May, A. (2002) Communities of practice: an opportunity for interagency working. *Journal of Clinical Nursing*, **11**, 394–398.

Lee-Baldwin, J. (2005) Asynchronous discussion forums: a closer look at the structure, focus and group dynamics that facilitate reflective thinking. *Contemporary Issues in Technology and Teacher Education*, **5**, 93–116

Lindahl, B. and Norberg, A. (2002) Clinical group supervision in an intensive care unit: a space for relief, and for sharing emotions and experiences of care. *Journal of Clinical Nursing*, **11**, 809–818.

Lindgren, B., Brulin, C., Holmlund, K. and Athlin, E. (2005) Nursing students' perception of group supervision during clinical training. *Journal of Clinical Nursing*, **14**, 822–829.

Maggs, C. and Biley, A. (2000) Reflections on the role of the nursing development facilitator in clinical supervision and reflective practice. *International Journal of Nursing Practice*, **6**, 192–195.

McGill, I. and Beaty, L. (2001) *Action Learning: A Guide for Professional, Management and Educational Development*, 2nd edn. Taylor Francis, Abingdon.

Mumford, A. (1996) Effective learners in action learning sets. *Journal of Workplace Learning*, **8**, 3–10.

Nursing and Midwifery Council (2004) *Code of Professional Conduct: Standards for Conduct, Performance and Ethics*. NMC, London.

Platzer, H. (2004) Are you sitting uncomfortably? From group resistance to group reflection in several uneasy moves. In: *Reflective Practice in Nursing* (eds C. Bulman and S. Schutz), 3rd edn. Blackwell Publishing, Oxford, pp. 113–127.

Platzer, H., Blake, D. and Ashford, D. (2000) Barriers to learning from reflection: a study of the use of groupwork with post-registration nurses. *Journal of Advanced Nursing*, **31**, 1001–1008.

Rolfe, G., Freshwater, D. and Jasper, M. (2001) *Critical Reflection for Nursing and the Helping Professions: A User's Guide*. Palgrave, Basingstoke.

Saarikoski, M., Warne, T., Aunio, R. and Leino-Kilpi, H. (2006) Group supervision in facilitating learning and teaching in mental health clinical placements: a case example of one student group. *Issues in Mental Health Nursing*, **27**, 273–285.

Sexton, L. (1999) Vicarious traumatisation of counsellors and effects on their workplaces. *British Journal of Guidance and Counselling*, **27**, 393–403.

Shanley, M.J. and Stevenson, C. (2006) Clinical supervision revisited. *Journal of Nursing Management*, **14**, 586–592.

Stark, S. (2006) Using action learning for professional development. *Educational Action Research*, **14**, 23–43.

Stevenson, C. (2005) Postmodernising clinical supervision in nursing. *Issues in Mental Health Nursing*, **26**, 519–529.

Walsh, K., Nicholson, J., Keough, C., Pridham, R., Kramer, M. and Jeffrey, J. (2003) Development of a group model of clinical supervision to meet the needs of a community mental health nursing team. *International Journal of Nursing Practice*, **9**, 33–39.

Wenger, E. (2000) Communities of practice and social learning systems. *Organization*, **7**, 225–246.

White, E. and Winstanley, J. (2006) Cost and resource implications of clinical supervision in nursing: an Australian perspective. *Journal of Nursing Management*, **14**, 628–636.

Chapter 6

Williams, B. and Walker, L. (2003) Facilitating perception and imagination in generating change through reflective practice groups. *Nurse Education Today*, **23**, 131–137.

Winship, G. and Hardy, S. (1999) Disentangling dynamics: group sensitivity and supervision. *Journal of Psychiatric and Mental Health Nursing*, **6**, 307–312.

Chapter 7

Using reflective journals and diaries to enhance practice and learning

Melanie Jasper

Introduction

Keeping a journal or diary is an activity that can be used for many different purposes. Indeed, there are numerous examples of authors documenting their experiences of living through events (e.g. Anne Frank), travelling in different parts of the world (e.g. Michael Palin), or as autobiography. This chapter will concentrate on journals used as a learning strategy to enable writers to reflect on and learn from the experiences they have and transform that learning into their own practice. It is intended as a practical chapter that provides tips and hints for using journal writing successfully and creatively in different contexts.

Many students will be using journals as part of course work, or to develop a learning log of evidence that they can draw from, to support a portfolio or to illustrate other forms of written work. More experienced practitioners may use journals to reflect on and explore events and incidents that have caused them to pause and think about their practice more deeply, so that their practice can be developed over time. Educators, whether working within a formal institution or in practice, are increasingly using learning journals to identify deep levels of learning and attempt to uncover how learners understand and apply theoretical concepts in a practice setting, or to provide evidence of a learner's progress towards learning objectives and outcomes. None of these examples of using journals are context free, as all students and practitioners will be working in the real world of health care, which is bound by codes of professional practice and standards of care that must be adhered to. I have included a section exploring ethical issues to be taken into consideration when using journal writing, especially as this may be used as a public document and seen by others.

What is a learning journal?

Many authors have debated the differences between the terms 'journal', 'diary' and 'log' (Holly 1988; Perkins 1996; Moon 1999a, 1999b), but essentially I am talking about a written record of experiences. This may simply be a chronological 'diary' of events such as we would use to organise our day, or may include the activity of 'journaling' which involves reflective writing about the events and experiences that we have had. In this chapter, I will use the term 'journal' to mean all of the types of writing that you may do that are reflective in nature and that are used to record your experiences on a continual basis. This is summarised very effectively by Thorpe (2004, p.325) who suggested that:

> 'Reflective learning journals refer to written documents that students (practitioners) create as they think about various concepts, events or interactions over a period of time for the purposes of gaining insights into self-awareness and learning'.

This draws attention to the notion of journal writing as essentially a strategy for learning from our experiences, and many claims have been made within the literature as to the effects of the processes of reflection used, within the medium of a journal. For instance, it is suggested that journal writing encourages the development of deeper levels of reflection (Blake 2005; Dye 2005; Walker 2006; Chirema 2007), whilst at the same time acknowledging that evidence of the more critical reflection expected at experienced practitioner level is often absent within reflective writing accounts (Thorpe 2004; Orland-Barak 2005; Chirema 2007).

Similarly, journal writing is said to enhance the development of critical thinking attributes such as the development of new understandings of situations, taking different perspectives on events and exploring alternative options for handling daily experiences (Williams et al. 2002; Fakude and Bruce 2003; Walker 2006), developing clinical reasoning (Kessler and Lund 2004; Kuiper 2004) and enhancing decision-making (Kuiper 2004). Other authors draw attention to the learning skills developed through the process of writing a journal, such as self-recognition of learning and learning needs (Knowlton et al. 2004; Dye 2005), transforming passive learners into active learners (Blake 2005; Dye 2005; Orland-Barak 2005), and prompting self-regulation and meta-cognition (Kuiper 2002). In short, journal writing is viewed as a valuable addition to the plethora of learning and teaching strategies available that specifically address the need for students to acknowledge learning from experiences within the context of professional practice.

Degazon and Lunney (1995) suggest that journal writing as a strategy for learning encompasses the tenets of adult education, in that:

- it proceeds at the learner's own pace;
- the learner selects the subject matter;
- it is an independent and solitary activity;
- there is freedom of expression, feelings, perceptions and frustrations without fear of exposure.

These points suggest that a journal needs to be under the control of the writer, who ultimately makes the decisions over its content, who else will see it, the style in which it is written and the way in which it is used. For a journal to be used for learning, it needs to have the following characteristics:

- It is compiled on an incremental basis over a period of time.
- It provides a record of events and experiences.
- It is focused on identifying learning that has occurred.
- It contains reflective commentaries or accounts.

(Jasper 2003)
These important characteristics are worth exploring in more detail.

The incremental basis of a journal

For a journal to document learning it needs to be built up incrementally over a period of time. This will show how the writer has grown and developed and worked his or her way towards achieving the learning outcomes that are expected. This is particularly so for students who need to develop to the level of professional competence within a set period of time and who have to, within that time, not only demonstrate theoretical and practical competence, but also develop the attributes of being a professional practitioner. This is often achieved through revisiting the original journal entry several times over a period of time, and reflecting anew on the experience. This enables writers to document their changing perceptions of the experience as they learn more, or see things differently, with the benefit of hindsight and further experience.

However, it is also becoming increasingly common for qualified nurses to use reflective journal writing within their professional portfolios, to demonstrate their on-going competence and learning throughout their practice. In fact, in a study exploring experienced nurses' use of reflective writing within portfolios, I found that the main reason nurses write reflectively is to provide evidence of their continuing competence through their careers (Jasper 1999). As with students' journals, particular aspects of a practitioner's development can be traced from the initial stimulus, such as an incident or event, through a series of reflections dedicated to developing learning and increasing understanding, which lead to changes in perception and behaviour, and professional, personal and practice development.

Chapter 7

Recording events and experiences

Not only is the journal an incremental record, but also it needs to be written *regularly*, so that it becomes a continual record of a person's experiences, or things that have happened to him/her. Of course, an expectation of daily entries is something only for the very committed! However, many practitioners find that they make entries in their journals when something happens that sticks in their minds and they feel the need to explore it in some detail through reflective strategies. To do this you need to write as full a description of the event as possible. This is important because our memory of events changes over time, and the version that we would write immediately after something has happened is likely to be very different from its description 3 or 6 months later. This is relevant to the assessment of reflection too. However, it is the detail in the immediacy of something that provides the basis for our learning, as it will include not simply an objective description of what has happened, but also our subjective *experience* of that event that is crucial to enabling us to understand the event in its entirety.

On-your-own exercise (20 minutes)

Why not test this out for yourself?

First of all, think back over the past few months and identify an event that has happened to you that you remember because of your emotional reactions to it. This might be something that made you very happy, gave you confidence in yourself, or represented some sort of achievement. Or, you might choose an event that made you angry, distressed or unhappy; or that left you feeling uncomfortable about the consequences. Write a description of this event in as much detail as you can remember.

It is likely that you have written a factual description of what happened, as if you are telling a story to someone else – is this true? If not, have you considered all angles in order to justify your conclusions?

Now think back to the event itself and attempt to recapture the feelings and emotions that you had at the time. Are these truly represented in the account that you have written? Can you identify the reasons for your answer?

Next time something happens that raises an emotional response in you, make a mental note to write it down as soon as possible after the event. Compare this description with the one that you made earlier and identify the differences.

These records of events and experiences build a picture of our lives as practitioners, and are fascinating as records of this in themselves. However, for journaling to be used as a tool for our learning, we need to be doing more than simply recording our experiences and initial reactions to them.

Identifying learning

It may be obvious to say that a *learning* journal needs to help writers identify their *learning*, but this is not quite as simple as it sounds. It is relatively easy to record achievements as a list, or to write a description of an experience and conclude with identifying what has been learnt as a result of it, but doing this within a journal is likely to involve a great deal more. First, you will be identifying your progress as your knowledge and skills develop over time. For instance, you may, as a student, have a book that records your skills in the practice environment, where you can see how you have progressed from a novice to being competent in the things you do. However, the entries relating to these skill acquisitions in your journal are likely to involve not only practical competence but also your growing awareness of the processes you are using to learn. This will include how you are learning, what you are learning, how you relate your previous knowledge to new experiences and how your knowledge is increasing as you progress through your course. These may comprise the ethical considerations regarding particular treatment activities that you undertake, or an awareness of the socio-economic constraints that inhibit certain groups from equal access to care, as well as the more practical elements of developing a skill and progressing to more complex nursing problems.

So whilst you can identify your learning through other mechanisms such as practice assessment documents, or examinations, the use of a learning journal is more likely to enable you to consider all the aspects of what happens to you. This helps you to consider it holistically, from different angles and outcomes, exploring differing solutions and resultant action that takes your learning from the theoretical to the practical.

Qualified practitioners may use journals to learn in a less formal or directive way, as they are not confined by course requirements. However, the processes being used are very similar, in that a learning journal becomes a record of the ways in which problems are identified and solved through reflective thinking and writing processes developed over time. This process is illustrated in Box 7.1 (although much of the detail has been removed from this extract), written by a student in order to demonstrate the developmental process that occurred.

This nurse, through revisiting the experience, changes her perceptions of the original event, enabling her to learn from it in a positive way. This is unlikely to have happened had she not used journaling to facilitate her thought processes and actively explore the total experience from different points of view. The ways in which this happens in journal writing is by the deliberate inclusion of reflective writing to help us to understand the processes of learning, and the wider issues involved.

Box 7.1   Reflections of a supervision group

Meeting one – we began the supervision group today, which is to last for two years. Having no prior experience of formal supervision I came to this as a novice, with a few feelings of trepidation but willing to go along with it as a new way of learning. Two incidents happened that stick out in my mind.

The initial task set for the group by the facilitator was to determine the ground rules that we would all sign up to. This resulted in the first confrontational dialogue between the tutor and certain members of the group. They challenged her style in determining the ground rules by writing on the blackboard what she thought the rules should be. I was beginning to feel uncomfortable, especially as the group was so small. We compromised by agreeing on having a general discussion, but delaying writing the rules until the next meeting when we could all be present.

The second incident that was particularly powerful for me was the group exercise that the tutor engaged us in. We were re-arranged to sit in a circle, eyes closed and asked to reveal our thoughts and make individual statements about how we felt. During this exercise, I could feel my anxiety rising and I desperately tried to disguise my true thoughts by delivering nondescript, unrevealing comments. I felt extremely vulnerable and annoyed at my docile acceptance of unquestioningly taking part in such an exercise. Certain members of the group again challenged the tutor as to the validity of such an exercise and abruptly ended it. It was their demonstrated experience and knowledge of such exercises that was a powerful learning event for me.

Reflection one week later – although I was shocked at my passivity, I realised that this was being driven by my profound sense of not being in control. I felt threatened and in a dependent position, and unable to get beyond the authority of the 'teacher'.

Three weeks later – this experience keeps coming back to me and reminds me of the many times in school and nurse training where I did what I was told, despite feeling uncomfortable and not wanting to conform. I realised the other day that this is because of the central role that authority figures, rules and approval have played in my life. I was a 'good' school child, and felt no need to challenge the systems and authority in what was a very didactic nurse education system. The apprenticeship model of training in the wards meant that you had to toe the line or you would get a 'bad' report. The hierarchical structure of nursing employment and grading reinforces this. So, whenever I am confronted with authority figures where

Contd.

I am not the one in control, I tend to do what I am told, despite feelings to the contrary. I wonder why I do this?

Two months later – we have now had two more group supervision sessions. I continue to feel extremely uncomfortable within these sessions and when I engage in discussion I remain reticent and thoughtful. Part of this is due to the conflicting messages given about the group. The way it is conducted is reminiscent of personal counselling, but in a group setting. My perception of group supervision was that we would learn new ways of thinking by viewing situations from multiple perspectives. These sessions do little to encourage critical thinking about practice development *per se*. Despite this negativity and concern, I am able to use my increased knowledge of group dynamics and my own behaviour in considering how I supervise those within my workplace. Through this, I now appreciate diverse reactions to supervision and the need for clear aims and focus in order to achieve practice development as opposed to personal problem solving.

Arising from the first experience I have made strong personal and professional relationships with three of the other members that have influenced my perspective on health care and our roles as nurses within it. They have fundamentally challenged my attitudes on group behaviour and reinforced my personal responsibility within this.

One year later – although I still smart at the memories of the first group, the bonding that occurred as a result of our joint negative experiences has actually turned into very strong relationships. I can see now what the facilitator was aiming to do, and in some ways can now sympathise with her position. I now have experiences of facilitating groups, and that first meeting is always anxiety provoking. It is very tempting to try to maintain control over the group by using exercises, but, as a result of my experiences, I never try to put the group members in this sort of position. I have learnt that, for me, the skilled facilitator is one who knows exactly which questions to ask, when to speak and when not, and how to manage group dynamics. Our own group has grown beyond what could possibly have been imagined in the first few meetings – in fact, it was doubtful whether people would actually turn up again! At the end of a year we have a strong group, offering support to each other and helping them to see ways through difficulties. Perhaps a little distress is needed in these groups for trust to occur – although I am still not convinced that confrontation is the most effective way to do it. For myself, I realise now that I have grown in terms of resisting the pull of the authority figure, and I am more assertive in situations that previously I would have deferred to another person because of their status.

Chapter 7

Reflective commentaries and accounts

The nature of reflective writing provides us with strategies for linking the experience itself with our learning. It is only by exploring our experiences in a reflective way that we will come to an understanding of the wider context of them, and just what and how we have learnt through them. In a way, reflective writing enables us to learn at a faster pace than if we were simply expecting to absorb knowledge and skills as we go through our course. This happens because we are consciously engaging in the process of writing as a learning tool in itself, and using it with the specific purpose of facilitating our learning. It is the *active* nature of reflection that enables us to acknowledge what we know, how we know it, what we do not know, and what we need to do to remedy this. The learning journal therefore provides the mechanism for not only linking theory with practice, but also *developing our own theories about practice for practice.*

Purposes of keeping a learning journal

Moon (1999b) presents 18 purposes for keeping a journal (summarised in Box 7.2).

If we look at these more closely, they can be grouped together under the following headings:

1. *Personal development – learning about oneself and one's practice*
   Learning journals are very personal and individual accounts of someone's journey at particular stages in their lives. The learning journal will incorporate not only the bare facts of events, but also the writer's experiences of those events, which will be different from those of anyone else that was there at the time. Hence, through using the journal, we learn about ourselves, the ways in which we react to things that happen to us, and our feelings about them. In Moon's (1999b) terms, this enhances our abilities to 'give voice' to this. The act of writing itself brings more to the learning process than simply recording the events. Below I summarise the features of reflective writing in relation to personal learning. In my book *Beginning Reflective Practice* (Jasper 2003) I wrote:

   'Writing helps us to:

   - Order our thoughts
   - Develop our analytical skills
   - Develop our critical thinking
   - Develop our creativity
   - Develop new understandings and knowledge

Box 7.2 The purposes of keeping learning journals (adapted from Moon 1999b, pp.189–193)

- To record experience
- To facilitate learning from experience
- To support understanding and the representation of the understanding
- To develop critical thinking or the development of a questioning attitude
- To encourage metacognition
- To increase active involvement in and ownership of learning
- To increase ability in reflection and thinking
- To enhance problem-solving skills
- As a means of assessment in formal education
- To enhance reflective practice
- For reasons of personal development and self-empowerment
- For therapeutic purposes or as a means of supporting behaviour change
- To enhance creativity
- To improve writing
- To improve or give 'voice'; as a means of self-expression
- To foster communication and foster reflective and creative interaction in a group
- To support planning and progress in research or a project
- As a means of communication between a learner and another

- Show us what we understand, and identifies the limits of our understanding.'

To these we can add Moon's criterion of problem-solving skills. These are all features that, once developed, will stay with us throughout our lives, and enable us to grow and move forward. These are often processes that we are unaware of because they are not tangible – we are unlikely to say that a particular event improved our critical thinking, for instance. However, the reflective activity that occurs in journal writing charts personal learning, serving to develop these attributes, which in turn are crucial to professional practice (Degazon and Lunney 1995).

On-your-own exercise (5 minutes)

Look back at the illustration in Box 7.1. Can you identify this nurse's personal development from her writing? Use the features of reflective writing identified above to organise your answers.

2. *Professional development*

   Every 3 years, registered nurses are required to provide evidence of continuing competence and accountability for their practice (NMC 2004b). To this end, nurses are expected to compile a personal profile or portfolio that details their continuing development over the previous 3 years. As I found in my own research, experienced nurses who use reflective writing within their portfolios did so primarily in order to provide evidence of their accountability as practitioners, in a way that was open to public scrutiny (Jasper 1999). Many of my respondents used journaling within their portfolios as a way of demonstrating their own increasing expertise and skill by providing detailed records of practice, professional and personal development. This might include, for instance, reflective activity relating to attendance at a study day, which resulted in evaluation of current practice, identification of where improvements could be made, piloting of new practices, further evaluation and readjustment, and so on. This shows that not only has an event been attended (which in itself does not indicate that anything has been learnt!) but also that the nurse understood the content, considered it in the light of her own practice, and applied it within a different context. Consequently journal writing is extremely useful in recording professional development because it provides not only the end result, but also, as with personal development, a record of the processes that the writer has gone through in order to achieve these.

3. *Facilitating learning*

   Several of Moon's purposes incorporate the notion of journaling as facilitating learning. Callister (1993) suggests that this enables the student to build a personal conceptual framework, with Haigh (2001) adding that journal writing makes students aware of the development of their learning and encourages them to recognise what is being learnt and how. Journal writing is a strategy primarily for experiential learning, i.e., the subject matter that is used arises from the writer's own experiences. It acts as a conduit between the *received* knowledge that we have (such as theoretical knowledge from external sources, or watching a practical skill) and the *applied* knowledge that results from considering the knowledge within a specific context. As Hahnemann (1986) suggests, journal writing is a process that forces students to search for connections and relationships in their learning.

4. *The development of reflective practice*

   Put simply, reflective practice involves completing the *experience–reflection–action* (ERA) cycle (Jasper 2003) that all models and frameworks propose. Reflective *practice* differs from simply engaging in reflection because it necessarily results in some action being taken –

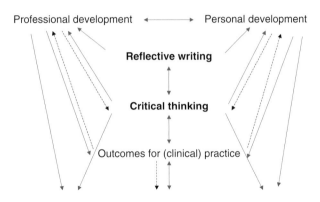

Developing a body of evidence of accountable practice

Fig. 7.1   Experienced nurses' use of reflective writing in portfolios (Jasper 2003, version two)

to 'practice' means to engage in practical activity, after all. This action might be very simple, such as deciding to go and look something up in the library, or it may be on a grander scale, such as initiating changes in practice resulting in practice development. The act and processes involved in journaling help the writer frame the action that will be taken as a result of reflecting on experiences, by drawing them through the reflective processes to conclusions focused on conscious action, behaviour and choice.

My updated model of the way experienced nurses use reflective writing in portfolios is presented in Fig. 7.1, and shows the links and relationships between the concepts proposed in my earlier model (Jasper 1999). These relationships are important in journaling, because they make explicit the significance of both the *processes* involved in writing reflectively and the *content* and *outcomes* that are its focus.

Styles of learning journals

There are many different types and variations on the style of journals, depending on the purpose they are being written for, who will have access to them and who will contribute to them. The key criterion for determining the most appropriate style of a journal is identifying the purpose for which the journal is being written. Once this has been established, the style of the journal follows on in a logical way.

The solitary journal

This type of journal is totally under the control of the writer, who makes all the decisions about its content, structure, purpose, style and use. Very often, the writer is choosing to keep a journal of this sort of his or her own volition. However, journals may also be used in courses where students are advised to write them for their own development, and to draw on these later, in assessed work. In the latter cases, the assessor will not be accessing the journal itself, but extracts from it will be used as evidence within the written assignments. An example of this style of journaling is given by Knowlton *et al.* (2004), who provide analysis and reflections on the effect of the journaling process on their individual development through a summary/reaction journal. They conclude that:

> '. . . writing the summary/reaction journals increased the amount of content that we learned and made our learning more durable'. (Knowlton *et al.* 2004, p.53)

This improvement in learning occurred in two ways: the summarising enabled writers to explain the content to themselves, and the writing enabled them to make connections between the course content and their own personal contexts. The authors suggest that it is the process of dialoguing with oneself that effects the improvement in learning as a result of the reflective writing process. There are, of course, other views; perhaps the most important is that dialoguing with oneself may result in reinforcement or affirmation of a standpoint rather than critical appraisal.

The 'writer-writes-reader-reads' journal

This style is most commonly found in student work, where students are required to keep a learning journal for some purpose specified by their course tutors. Hence the student writes and the lecturer/assessor reads and may make comments in feedback. The amount of control the writer has in this style can vary a great deal. At one extreme, students are given the journal format, told what they need to write in it and given structures such as a reflective model or framework to be used and the types of reflective components required, such as learning contracts, critical incident analyses, diaries or logs and reflective reviews. Various examples of journals of this sort are summarised in Table 7.1.

Journals used for other purposes, such as those used by practitioners in compiling professional portfolios, will clearly be more loosely structured than those where large numbers of students are required to complete them for assignment purposes and standardisation is required. Although the *PREP* (NMC 2004b) regulations necessitate a portfolio being kept, the content of it is left up to the nurse, providing it shows that the required components to demonstrate competence have been

Table 7.1   Some journaling strategies

Author(s)	Journaling strategy
Cook (2000)	Recorded experiences throughout the course, including lectures, reading and clinical work. These were reflected on and made sense of in terms of their own learning
Cooper and Taft (2005)	Nursing students in final clinical experience wrote 'thinking-in-action' reflections during online clinical conferences. Students' reflections were used to inform nursing faculty about issues affecting students' preparation for professional practice
Dye (2005)	Self-S.O.A.P. (subjective, objective, assessment, action plan) notes used with physical therapy students and submitted to clinical educators. Feedback aimed at promoting further reflection
Grant et al. (2006)	Voluntary use of reflective journals by medical students. Feedback in discussion groups. Participants gained a greater ability to identify learning objectives and integrate learning. No difference in examination results between the groups
Kessler and Lund (2004)	Weekly online journal used in distance learning approach, with feedback, guidance and support provided by faculty each week
King and LaRocco (2006)	e-journaling through a virtual learning environment in two graduate level courses, and interactive journals between course participant and instructor
Maloney and Campbell-Evans (2002)	Student-teachers used journal entries to get direction on practice and planning, as a tool for analysis and as an emotional release
Marland and McSherry (1997)	Students spent 30 minutes at the end of each shift reviewing and recording their personal experiences and observations. Entries used in tutorial and group discussions, as well as for individual feedback
Milinkovic and Field (2005)	Reflective journal used by undergraduate radiation therapy students to document clinical experiences. Feedback by clinical academic on their reflective skills and in helping students to learn and become reflective practitioners
Simpson and Courtney (2007)	Journal through a clinical practicum to foster development of critical thinking. This enabled the creation of dialogue between nurse educators and nurses
Swindell and Watson (2006)	Development of ethical practice in social work students through self-reflective journaling in a 45-minute classroom session. Educator feedback given

achieved. For the purposes of audit, any journal kept by a nurse will not be considered as part of the profile that needs to be seen by a reviewer.

The dialogue journal

Drevdahl and Dorcy (2002) and Maloney and Campbell-Evans (2002) provide examples of journals used as a form of communication between the student and teacher where a dialogue style is used. Drevdahl and Dorcy (2002) call this style 'conversing in writing' in which students are encouraged to write about their experiences, ask questions, and share thoughts that they might not want to verbalise. It keeps the teacher abreast of the student's experiences, and provides a forum through which the teacher can reply to the student's writing on an on-going basis and vice versa.

Hurtig et al. (1989) call this style an *interactive* journal because a daily record of the student's 'ideas, feelings, actions and reactions that relate to a nursing practicum' is created, to which the teacher responds. This creates a diary that is an interaction between student and teacher. This enables teaching to be individualised, and the student to receive immediate and on-going feedback, with learning deficits identified and remedied swiftly.

Another example of this is where practitioners set up dialogue journals between themselves as a way of bouncing ideas around and learning from each other's reflectivity and experiences. With the use of the internet and email, and the abundance of focused chat rooms available, this is a growing way for a journal to be used and contributed to by more than one person (e.g. Driscoll and Townsend 2007).

The group journal

The dialogue journal can be developed beyond two people to include teamwork and group discussion. It is particularly useful for developmental situations where group projects are undertaken or new ideas and processes are being tested (e.g. Alterio 2004). In action research situations, for instance, where all members of a team are testing new ways of working, an on-going journal that everyone has access to and where you can record your thoughts or ideas on a daily basis is a very useful way of capturing the everyday experiences and insights that may be crucial to the success of the project. Although this can happen through paper-based records, the development of on-line facilities makes this a useful and instant way of creating the dialogue.

Another way in which group journals can be used in patient settings is for team members to record case diaries detailing different perspectives and developments in a patient's care. This is different to case notes because there is freedom for subjective feelings and experiences to be recorded and shared with other members of the team.

Clearly, there are many creative and innovative ways that journals can be structured to meet the needs of the person writing and the type of event that is being reflected on. The choice of which approach to use is often dependent upon the content of the journal itself, and it is to this that I now turn.

The content of the journal

As a private document, a journal can include whatever you want it to. There are no rules about personal reflective writing – the important thing is to use it to achieve the purpose you are using it for, and to write it in a way you want to write it. So, where there are no rules, the scope for variety and innovation is very broad. Below I present various ways in which you might write reflectively, from the straightforward descriptive account, to those that are more creative or analytical. It is worth experimenting with different styles of writing, selecting those that suit your learning style and the type of event, experience or incident that you are exploring. Suggestions for different types of writing activities that may be used in a journal can be found in Table 7.2.

Rolfe *et al.* (2001) grouped writing into analytical and creative strategies as a useful way of dividing those that may be outcome driven and those that may be more directed at exploring emotions and feelings. In using analytical strategies, we focus on using our experiences as objective data that we can analyse to identify our learning. These techniques are most likely to be used where other people are likely to read the journal. *Critical incident analyses* and using *structured frameworks for reflection*, for instance, help us to stand back from our own experiences of the event, using analysis and critique to arrive at different perceptions. Many of these may take a great deal of time to complete effectively and may not be suitable for everyday use and thus are reserved for specific incidents. However, Borton's (1970) framework, which simply asks questions directed through three question stems, is an easy framework to carry in your head and use on an everyday basis. Box 7.3 shows how these stems can be used to focus your reflective writing. The question examples given are only provided as illustrations and you do not need to remember these – the important point is to memorise the 'What?', 'So what?' 'Now what?' phrases so that they can be used to structure your reflective work.

Other techniques are even quicker and easier to use, and can enable you to work with your journal as a 'friend'. For instance, the *three-a-day* technique asks you to simply write a record of your day/experience, etc. and identify three aspects of learning that have been achieved. This might simply be 'Three things I have learnt today are . . .', to more complex ideas such as 'Three things I need to find out more about are . . .' or 'Three things that I need to do as a result of this are. . . .'

Chapter 7

Table 7.2   Reflective writing strategies

Analytical strategies	Creative strategies
• Critical incident analyses • Dialogical writing (creating a conversation through questions and answers) • Making a case – exploring the alternative perspectives of an issue • Creating an on-going record • Exploring a problem • SWOT[1] analysis • Using a structured reflective framework, e.g. Rolfe *et al.* (2001); Johns (2004) in Johns and Freshwater (2005) • Identifying three-a-day, e.g. 'Three things I have learnt from this shift are . . .' or 'Three tips for future practice from this experience are . . .'. These can be varied to ensure that the learning strategy is varied and does not become stale • Page-a-day record of experiences • Writing a word limited summary • Identifying specific aspects from a situation, e.g. focusing on knowledge, or skills analysis • Learning outcomes – using these as reflective cues to review an experience • Identifying competencies	• Writing the unsent letter (or email) • Writing to a nominated other person, e.g. your mother or a close friend • Writing as the other person • Writing as a journalist • Storytelling/fantasy • Poetry • Creating a review in a particular style

[1] A strategy that involves identifying the strengths, weaknesses, opportunities and threats within an experience.

Finally, there are the techniques that ask us to analyse our experience against given objectives such as providing evidence of pre-specified *learning outcomes* or *identifying competencies*. These enable us to focus on what we are trying to achieve by working backwards from an end point. It may be that you want to build up a record of your own competency development over the length of your course – in which case separate journal pages for each competency would be a useful and effective structure. Alternatively, you might want to work on developing the evidence base to support learning outcomes for modules you are studying, using your reflective journal as resource material when you are writing an assignment or compiling a portfolio of evidence. The advantages of working towards specific objectives are that you know what it is that you

Box 7.3   Borton's (1970) framework used to guide nursing reflective activity

What?	So what?	Now what?
This is the descriptive level, and all the questions that are asked start with the word what	At this level we look deeper at what is going on behind the experience, to explore it at a theoretical and conceptual level	Building on the previous level, these questions enable us to consider alternative courses of action and choose the most appropriate
Example	**Example**	**Example**
What happened? What did I do? What did others do? What did I feel? What was I trying to achieve? What was good or bad about the experience?	So what is the importance of this? So what is the significance of this for me? So what more do I need to know about this? So what have I learnt about this?	Now what could I do? Now what would be the best thing to do? Now what do I need to do? Now what will I do? Now what might be the consequences of this action?

are aiming for, and can draw up action plans for achieving these. You can also decide what evidence it is that you will need to demonstrate them in a planned and incremental way, and through using the journal, constantly review how far you have progressed.

Creative techniques, on the other hand, are very individualistic and it is unlikely that these would be used where the writing was required as a course component and going to be read by others, unless the writer chooses to share it. *Letter or email writing* in its many forms is a useful strategy for recording emotional experiences, where writers need to rid themselves of tension before dealing with an incident. *Writing the unsent letter*, for instance, enables writers to record their feelings as if writing to the person who has instigated them. Often this strategy enables a distance to be created, because the emotional aspects are poured onto the paper, allowing the person to be more rational in dealing with the incident itself. One word of caution with this idea though – when using email to vent your feelings, take care not to push the 'send' button! *Writing with another person in mind* again allows specific viewpoints to be taken, where writers can defend their position without contradiction, whereas *writing as the other* forces writers to consider alternative ways of experiencing the event. This can be a useful exercise if you are finding it difficult to get beyond your own emotional responses to something that has happened and need to find a way out of your thought patterns.

Journalist writing, story telling and poetry writing all enable writers to be creative in sifting through the contents of the experience, reforming it in a different way that helps them to make sense of it and get to the nub of what may be bothering them about it. For instance, imagine yourself as Alaistair Cooke writing a *Letter from America* or as Jon Snow sending a broadcast back from a distant land to the television. Or perhaps consider how Harry Potter would have dealt with that difficult character!

For most of us, the inclination is to simply sit down and start writing a description of an event in a linear form. Others may prefer the order imposed on our thoughts by using a reflective framework that guides us through specific cues in order to explore an incident. Once you have been writing a journal for some time you will find a strategy that suits you best and that you are comfortable with. However, the suggestions and alternatives above provide examples of how others have used variety in their writing, and devised ways of keeping the journal fresh and dynamic. It may be worth considering experimenting with some of these and seeing what the results are.

This classification is obviously a simplistic one, and is not meant to suggest that the strategies exist in isolation. Indeed, any action will have emotions and feelings associated with it. I have divided them in this way as an illustration of the different foci and outcomes that we might take in our reflective writing, and to emphasise that we can choose from a whole range of ideas depending on what it is we want to achieve and get out of the activity. They provide us with a 'kitbag' of tools that we can select from as appropriate for the jobs that we want them to do.

On-your-own exercise (10 minutes)

Think about each of the reflective writing strategies in Table 7.2 in turn and answer the following questions.

- What is my initial reaction to this technique – positive, negative, appealing, offputting, comfortable or uncomfortable?
- Why might this be?
- In what ways could I use this technique?
- What sorts of events and experiences within my practice could I use this technique for?
- How could I incorporate strategies for reflective practice within the technique?

Getting started in journal writing

Having thought about what you will write about, and how you will approach writing, the next task is to get started. Unfortunately there is no enlightening advice I can offer about how to start writing. It seems churlish to say 'Just sit down and do it', but that is simply how it is! However, there are various strategies that you can adopt to help motivate yourself to write:

1. It is important to identify your own reasons for wanting to keep a journal, especially if it is not something that you are required to do as part of a course. Look again at the purposes of keeping a journal in Box 7.2 and try to identify those that apply to you. Understanding your motivation, and perhaps writing a reflective piece exploring why you feel the desire to keep a journal, can be the first step to actually starting it (and may be the first piece of writing that goes in the journal!).

2. Identifying your attitudes to writing and where these have come from may free you from the rules and boundaries inhibiting your writing.

3. Establishing a comfortable environment in which to write helps to link writing with relaxation and taking control of the situation. For instance, are you more comfortable writing on a computer than with a pen and paper; or maybe you like to write with a special pen and notebook, or in a particular place? Perhaps you need to have completed the rest of your daily activities and use specific times in the day to write? Try to think about how you can create an environment to suit yourself that will allow you to start writing.

4. Identify previous enjoyable experiences of writing and plan to use the elements of these that made them pleasurable. These might be types of writing that you liked (e.g. structured/unstructured, task driven/ free flowing) and work out how you can plan to use these in your journal. Often, the barriers we put up against starting to write derive from previous experiences that we found stressful, such as examinations or writing essays from our school days.

5. Plan to start simply – perhaps set yourself a target of writing a certain number of words a day, or use the 'three-a-day' technique to review your day and identify significant events and experiences that have happened. Gradually plan to expand what you are doing, and how you are doing it, as you become more comfortable with writing and confident of what you are achieving.

Chapter 7

Structuring a journal

At some stage you will need to consider how your journal is going to be organised. At first you may be content to write in a linear fashion, page by page. However, there are other ways in which a diary can be organised, which will facilitate reflective activity and enable you to return to entries and add to your thought processes and learning over time. Some of these are summarised in Table 7.3.

Again, the decisions about the structure of your journal need to arise from your knowledge about yourself – your learning and writing style, the way you motivate yourself and the ways in which you achieve your objectives in other parts of your life. Try to incorporate these into the structure of your journal, as you are more likely to succeed if you are using familiar tried and tested ways that you are comfortable with, and use them to start your journal.

Ethical issues

Unless required for course work, journals tend to be very private documents. Journaling is under the control of the writer, and a deliberate decision needs to be taken if the entries are to be seen by others. This is not to be undertaken lightly, as many of the entries will be of experiences that have emotional significance attached to them for the writer, and/or may be records of incidents where professional misconduct or incidents of questionable quality of care may be recorded.

Nurses are bound by their Code of Professional Conduct (NMC 2004a) for the whole period of time that they are recorded on the live register of nurses, midwives and health visitors. Thus the decision to show journal entries to others must be taken in the knowledge that professional consequences may ensue if the Code of Conduct has been contravened. Of course, no-one can make you reveal any part of your journal or professional portfolio to others. Where it is required to be a public document, you have the choice of what is included in the public part and can remove anything that may result in negative consequences for yourself.

Also, do remember that most of the people you will be sharing your journal with will be in a position of authority and are likely to be nurses. Therefore they also have a professional responsibility within the Code of Conduct and may feel the need to take further action about something you have written. They may also facilitate you to consider your own actions and encourage you to seek alternatives or develop what you have done.

Finally, do also remember the need for confidentiality and anonymity regarding any other person that has a part in your journal. This applies to anyone else – patients and their carers, professional workers,

Table 7.3   Some techniques for structuring your journal

Structure/technique	How it works
The open-page technique	The pages of the book are opened out so the two pages are used for each event/experience. The full description is written on the left-hand page in as much detail as possible. The right-hand page is used for reflective activity. The entries are dated, starting with the initial reflection. The pages are returned to at intervals (possibly on a completely random basis), with new reflections being added incrementally, thus developing new insights as the incident itself recedes into the background
The revolving spiral	This involves exploring an incident using a reflective cycle, such as Borton's (1970) or Gibbs et al. (1988) framework for reflection, and creating a reflective review of an incident. The outcome of this will be a changed perspective and probable action that will be taken. Hence, the next time a similar experience occurs it can be explored using the same process, thus creating a continuous spiral of learning through developing expertise and perceptions of a single topic
Organising a journal through a framework	This is most common when a journal is part of course work and students need to demonstrate learning outcomes such as competencies or a range of experience. Sections can be created for each of these, within which cues are used to facilitate the reflective writing. For instance, students may use a framework to identify their previous learning and knowledge about a topic, resulting in the identification of specific learning needs, a plan of action to achieve these, identification of the evidence that will be used to support their achievement, and a reflective review of the process
Focused topic areas	This technique is used where a specific topic is focused on in order to structure the learning to be achieved. Each section in the journal relates to one topic, and is revisited on a regular basis
Project/research journals and diaries	These are used specifically to keep an on-going reflective log of the progress of a project or research study. They enable the researcher to record memos, analytical notes and ideas as the project progresses and develops, thus creating an audit trail

Chapter 7

colleagues and educational staff. If you are in any doubt about this, try not to use other people's names at all, or if you do, give them pseud-onyms and make this clear at the beginning of the journal. Another issue to consider that is related to this is the use of patient information as evidence or in illustration of your work. Do remember that the Data Protection Act (1998) applies to you, and if you are unclear about your responsibilities within this legislation it is worth checking this out.

On-your-own exercise (20 minutes)

Think about the issues raised in this section in relation to creating your own journal:

- What aspects of the Code of Professional Conduct do you need to consider when starting your journal?
- Who are you going to be sharing your journal with, and what are the implications of this?
- How would you ensure that you maintained confidentiality and anonymity?
- Do you need to know more about the Data Protection Act (1998), and if so, what are you going to do about it?

Using journals as an educator

As with any teaching and learning strategy, it is in the planning that the grounds for success or failure are laid. Using journaling to facilitate learning needs to be part of the overall strategy to facilitate the professional development of the student. It is clear that where journaling is used within courses in addition to formalised assessment strategies, students are unlikely to give it as much time and effort as where it is part of the assessment process (Grant *et al.* 2006; Walker 2006). However, the benefits of journaling in terms of enabling students to understand their own learning and in facilitating deep learning are also clearly documented above. Hence, the educator needs to establish a clear rationale and process for using journaling with students if it is to achieve the outcomes for students that are anticipated.

In Box 7.4 I pass on some tips for using journaling that I have learnt over the years. I hope that these may aid anyone contemplating using journaling in their own teaching practice, and that they may help prevent the pitfalls that both I and others writing in the literature have encountered in the past.

Box 7.4   Facilitating others to use journals

Teacher credibility

Ensure that you are clear about:

- why you are asking the student to keep a journal;
- your own attitudes towards journaling;
- the purpose you want it to serve;
- the outcomes you expect it to achieve;
- how it will be used as part of your learning and teaching strategy;
- the ethical issues involved.

A question to think about:

- Is it ethical to ask students to keep a journal if you don't do so yourself?

The nuts and bolts

Think about:

- what type of structure you want the students to use, or whether to leave this to the student;
- what the journal will be used for, e.g. assessment, individual tutorials, group work;
- how to ensure it will be at the appropriate academic level for the module/course;
- whether it is compulsory;
- the style of journal you are using;
- whether it is formative or summative;
- how you are going to assess it;
- what you are going to assess;
- how you can make the marking as straightforward as possible;
- whether your marking criteria are appropriate for this type of assessment tool;
- whether you will ask the student to self-assess;
- whether others are to be involved, e.g. mentors, in either writing, assessing or both.

Contd.

Chapter 7

Student preparation

It is worth taking time to:

- Prepare detailed student notes
- Spend a couple of hours briefing the students
- Prepare exemplars and illustrations
- Prepare exercises based on different types of experiences/events
- Prepare exercises using different writing strategies
- Discuss the ethical issues
- Identify what it is you are expecting from students and how it relates to their other work/course outcomes.

Teaching and learning strategies

- It is worth using a learning contract that is negotiated between yourself and the student in terms of outcomes, objectives, structure, action planning and strategies to be used
- Allocate time for individual tutorials so that you can be sure the student understands what is expected of them
- Plan group tutorials/seminars for students to share their experiences of using the journal
- Plan regular review time to ensure that students are using the journal incrementally
- Create milestones so that students have something to aim for, e.g. three a day exercises, monthly 500 word summaries, etc.
- Establish sound strategies for process and content of feedback to the student
- Create strategies for self-assessment.

NB: Time spent at the beginning in facilitating and supporting students pays dividends at the end!

Conclusion

This chapter has, by necessity, provided a very broad and wide-ranging overview of the use of journals as a learning strategy. It is hoped that students and qualified practitioners alike will be stimulated to try a version of journaling themselves within their professional lives. For many of the nurses I have worked with, the act of journaling brought reflective practice alive and made it, if not an everyday conscious activity, then certainly a regular one. Many have found that journaling enabled them to see the task of constructing a professional portfolio as a dynamic activity, rather than an onerous, retrospective, dust-gathering chore. So, why not try it yourself and see?

References

Alterio, M. (2004) Collaborative journaling as a professional development tool. *Journal of Further and Higher Education*, **28** (3), 321–332.

Blake, T.K. (2005) Journaling: an active learning technique. *International Journal of Nursing Education Scholarship*, **2** (1), article 7.

Borton, T. (1970) *Reach, Touch, and Teach*. McGraw-Hill, London.

Callister, L.C. (1993) The use of student journals in nursing education: making meaning out of clinical experience. *Journal of Nursing Education*, **32** (4), 185–186.

Chirema, K.D. (2007) The use of reflective journals and learning in post-registration nursing students. *Nurse Education Today*, **27**, 192–202.

Cook, I. (2000) 'Nothing can ever be the case of "Us" and "Them" again': exploring the politics of difference through border pedagogy and student journal writing. *Journal of Geography in Higher Education*, **24** (1), 13–27.

Cooper, C. and Taft, L.B. (2005) Preparing for practice: students' reflections on their final clinical experience. *Journal of Professional Nursing*, **21** (5), 293–302.

Degazon, C.E. and Lunney, M. (1995) Clinical journal: a tool to foster critical thinking for advanced levels of competence. *Clinical Nurse Specialist*, **9** (5), 270–274.

Drevdahl, D.J. and Dorcy, K.S. (2002) Using journals for community health students engaged in group work. *Nurse Educator*, **27** (6), 255–259.

Driscoll, J. and Townsend, A. (2007) Alternative methods in clinical supervision: beyond the face-to-face encounter. In: *Practising Clinical Supervision: A Reflective Approach for Healthcare Professionals* (ed. J. Driscoll). Baillière Tindall, Elsevier, Edinburgh.

Dye, D. (2005) Enhancing critical reflection of students during a clinical internship using the Self-S.O.A.P. note. *Internet Journal of Allied Health Sciences and Practice*, **3** (4), http://ijahsp.nova.edu.

Fakude, L.P. and Bruce, J.C. (2003) Journaling: a quasi-experimental study of student nurses' reflective learning ability. *Curationis*, **26** (2), 49–55.

Gibbs, G., Farmer, B. and Eastcott, D. (1988) *Learning by Doing. A Guide to Teaching and Learning Methods*. FEU, Birmingham Polytechnic.

Grant, A., Kinnersley, P., Metcalf, E., Pill, R. and Houston H. (2006) Students' views of reflective learning techniques: an efficacy study at a UK medical school. *Medical Educator*, **40**, 379–388.

Hahnemann, B.K. (1986) Journal writing: a key to promoting critical thinking in nursing students. *Journal of Nursing Education*, **25** (5), 213–215.

Haigh, M.J. (2001) Constructing Gaia: using journals to foster reflective learning. *Journal of Geography in Higher Education*, **25** (2), 167–189.

Holly, M.L. (1988) Reflective writing and the spirit of enquiry. *Cambridge Journal of Education*, **19** (1), 71–80.

Hurtig, W., Yonge, O., Bodnar, D. and Berg, M. (1989) The interactive journal: a clinical teaching tool. *Nurse Educator*, **14** (6), 17, 31, 35.

Jasper, M. (1999) Assessing and improving student outcomes through reflective writing. In: *Improving Student Learning Outcomes* (ed. C. Rust), Chapter 1. Oxford Centre for Staff Development, Oxford.

Jasper, M. (2003) *Beginning Reflective Practice*. Nelson Thornes, Cheltenham.

Johns, C. and Freshwater, D. (2005) *Transforming Nursing Through Reflective Practice*, 2nd edn. Blackwell Publishing, Oxford.

Kessler, P.D. and Lund, C.H. (2004) Reflective journaling: developing an online journal for distance education. *Nurse Educator*, **29** (1), 20–24.

King, F.B. and LaRocco, D.J. (2006) E-journaling: a strategy to support student reflection and understanding. *Current Issues in Education*, **9** (4), http://cie.ed.asu.edu/volume9/number 4.

Knowlton, D.S., Eschmann, A., Fish, N., Heffren, B. and Voss, H. (2004) Processes and impact of journal writing in a graduate-level theory course: students' experiences and reflections. *Teaching and Learning*, **18** (2), 43–56.

Kuiper, R.A. (2002) Enhancing metacognition through the reflective use of self-regulated learning strategies. *Journal of Continuing Education in Nursing*, **33**, 78–87.

Kuiper, R.A. (2004) Nursing reflections from journaling during a perioperative internship. *AORN Journal*, **79** (1), 195–218.

Maloney, C. and Campbell-Evans, G. (2002) Using interactive journal writing as a strategy for professional growth. *Asia-Pacific Journal of Teacher Education*, **30** (1), 39–50.

Marland, G. and McSherry, W. (1997) The reflective diary: an aid to practice-based learning. *Nursing Standard*, **12**, 13–15, 49–52.

Milinkovic, D. and Field, N. (2005) Demystifying the reflective clinical journal. *Radiography*, **11**, 175–183.

Moon, J. (1999a) *Learning Journals*. Kogan Page, London.

Moon, J. (1999b) *Reflection in Learning and Professional Development*. Kogan Page, London.

Nursing and Midwifery Council (2004a) *Code of Professional Conduct: Standards for Conduct, Performance and Ethics*. NMC, London.

Nursing and Midwifery Council (2004b) *The PREP Handbook*. NMC, London.

Orland-Barak, L. (2005) Portfolios as evidence of reflective practice: what remains untold. *Educational Research*, **47** (1), 25–44.

Perkins, J. (1996) Reflective journals: suggestions for educators. *Journal of Physical Therapy Education*, **10** (1), 8–13.

Rolfe, G., Freshwater, D. and Jasper, M. (2001) *Critical Reflection for Nursing and the Helping Professions: A User's Guide*. Palgrave, Basingstoke.

Simpson, E. and Courtney, M. (2007) A framework for guiding critical thinking through reflective journal documentation: a Middle Eastern experience. *International Journal of Nursing Practice*, **13**, 203–208.

Swindell, M.L. and Watson, J. (2006) Teaching ethics through self-reflective journaling. *Journal of Social Work Ethics and Values*, **3** (2), http://www.socialworker.com/jswve/content/view/37/46/.

Thorpe, K. (2004) Reflective learning journals: from concept to practice. *Reflective Practice*, **5** (3), 327–343.

Walker, S.E. (2006) Journal writing as a teaching technique to promote reflection. *Journal of Athletic Training*, **41** (2), 216–221.

Williams, R.M., Wessel, J., Gemus, M. and Foster-Sargeant, E. (2002) Journal writing to promote reflection by physical therapy students during clinical placements. *Physiotherapy Theory and Practice*, **18** (1), 5–15.

Chapter 8

Continuing the journey with reflection

Sue Duke

I start this third episode of my journey with reflection with an entry from my reflective journal. The other two episodes were told in the previous two editions of this book (Duke 2000, 2004). This entry summarises my experience of caring for a person that I have named Kate, whilst a nurse consultant in palliative care in an acute hospital. This record of my experience will be used throughout the chapter to reflect upon the issues I raised in the previous two episodes and to portray how my journey has subsequently developed.

Extract from my reflective diary, April 2003:

> Kate was a 67 year old woman with a brain tumour. She had been referred to me for symptom management and ongoing care planning. She was experiencing dizziness on movement and associated vomiting and had a left leg weakness. This challenged her ability to be independent and influenced her ability to sleep. Up until recently Kate had had a part time job and helped to care for two grandchildren. Over the time that I had been seeing her we had managed to minimise her symptoms and although Kate really wanted to get home as soon as possible, we had discussed the possibility of a hospice admission for rehabilitation. Although initially reluctant Kate had agreed that it would be better to go home more independent than go home and struggle. I asked the palliative medicine consultant to see Kate with the view of offering her a bed. When I introduced her to the consultant Kate put her hand up to her head and said to the consultant, 'Please excuse my hair, it has not been done for a while. I usually have it done each week. I expect it looks a mess'. The consultant assured her it was fine and moved on in her assessment to explore Kate's symptoms and how she felt about coming to the hospice. Throughout the assessment Kate kept her hand over her head as though she was trying to hide her hair.
>
> I stayed with Kate after the consultant had gone and asked her if she would like me to wash her hair. Kate explained that she

would be too dizzy having this done and would be likely to vomit again. I said that we could do this for her in bed and that she would not need to do anything other than lie flat. She gave me a very steady look, smiled and agreed. I went to find a colleague to help me and after about 30 minutes we had washed and dried Kate's hair, given her a blanket bath and changed her sheets and she was fast asleep.

Introduction

This is not the first time that I have written about the experience of washing a patient's hair in bed. It is something that I really enjoy – I like the morale boost it provides to people unable to get out of bed, and the paraphernalia involved in achieving this. For me there is a contradiction within this process that points to the knowledge of nursing and as a consequence sustains me as a nurse. This contradiction is about an ordinary everyday activity, undertaken by all of us and by other professionals (such as hairdressers), that becomes transformed into an extraordinary activity, not by the situation in which it takes place (although in bed is a fairly extraordinary place to have your hair washed) but by the nursing knowledge inherent in this process. This is the rub of course. I claim that there is nursing knowledge within this process, but I find it difficult to articulate the knowledge involved; the aesthetic, personal and spiritual nature of this knowledge defying my abilities to adequately express it in words. Yet I continue to try and this effort is the focus of the chapter. The chapter will track the development of this effort, my continuing journey with reflection as I try to articulate my knowledge, the motivations underpinning this endeavour and the relationship between this knowledge and my identity as a nurse.

This exploration is organised by differing points in my journey in finding ways of articulating my practice: hidden nursing – the quest to articulate palliative care nursing; missing nursing – treating nursing as an event rather than as a process; subverting nursing – the dangers of academic form and the rhetoric of evidence-based practice; reflecting nursing – examining my reflective voice; and portraying nursing – redefining my reflective voice. My reflection of caring for Kate is used to provide examples of this journey and is re-examined in the second part of the chapter in order to assess how it influences and fits with my understanding of nursing.

Hidden nursing – the quest to articulate palliative care nursing

The first time I published a story of hair-washing I wrote of my experience with Doris, a patient I cared for early in my appointment as a Lecturer

Practitioner in Palliative Care. Caring for Doris was one of four stories that I wrote as exemplars for a paper on hidden nursing I co-authored (Duke and Copp 1992). The thrust of the paper was the importance of articulating nursing and asserting its value to mitigate a reductionist approach to care. We ended the article by stating that as nurses we must 'describe what we are doing and, most of all, value our contribution to patient care' (p.42). The motivation to articulate palliative care nursing came at a time when palliative medicine was developing as a speciality. The knowledge inherent in symptom management was being given more importance compared to other less tangible aspects of care, such as psychological and spiritual care. I felt as though much of my experience in palliative care was being devalued, that it counted for little if it was not to do with helping others to manage people's symptoms.

Articulating the hidden, intangible aspects of my care became a quest that I embraced to counter the emphasis placed on empirical knowledge and the medical voice. Although not the reason that I started to use reflection (rather I stumbled into it as a consequence of thinking that 'I better have a go' as I had designed an assessment strategy based around reflection for the students I was about to teach), it became a means by which I could enact this quest. Frank (1995) describes a quest as a search for an alternative way – in his discussion, an alternative way of being ill; in mine, an alternative way to understanding nursing. I wrote reflections of my practice as carefully as I could in order to capture the skill of my practice, trying to craft a story that stood for nursing.

However, as I described in the second edition of this book (Duke 2000), I rarely analysed my accounts of practice. Paradoxically this meant that I did not articulate the knowledge embedded within them and rarely drew on them to develop my understanding of practice. Instead I treated them as having an inherent salience, almost as if they were sacred artefacts of my practice. As a consequence, my reflection was more anecdotal and indulgent than educative about nursing. As argued by Paley and Eva (2005) in relation to health care narratives in general, they tended to romanticise my practice through emotional persuasiveness rather than by careful evaluation. Nevertheless, they were important in helping me to describe my practice and this was a first step in becoming skilled in reflection.

The next step in the development of my ability to reflect and in my endeavour to portray nursing involved analysing descriptions of my expe-rience by considering differing kinds of knowledge that might explain my practice – aesthetic, empirical, ethical, personal and socio-contextual. This not only helped me to develop the range and depth of my knowl-edge but also enabled me to make connections across the varying kinds of practice that I was engaged in, particularly between clinical, education and management practice. As a consequence I was able to integrate the differing kinds of practice that were inherent in my lecturer practitioner role and to be more effective. In short, I had begun to reflect in the way described by Boyd and Fales (1983, p.100). This process resulted in 'changes in conceptual perspective'. I began to view my experience as a means by which I could learn more about my practice. Experience became central to my learning, as Boud *et al.* (1993, p.8) suggest, and I began to learn how it needed to be 'arrested, examined, analysed, considered and negated to shift it to knowledge' (Aitchison and Graham 1989, p.15). I also learnt that I was central to this process. I learnt that reflection 'created and clarified meaning in terms of self' (Boyd and Fales 1983, p.100) and that I had to actively engage in the process in order to examine my assumptions and draw new meanings from my practice experience (Brookfield 1996).

This process was not without its dangers. The endeavour of seeking knowledge to explain my practice invited an end result. Reflection sometimes became a quest for an adequate explanation that in some ways completed the experience, wrapped up the ends and packaged up the experience into an account that was inclusive of differing sources of knowledge. This is a poor use of experience. It treats it as if it is an event, something that happened rather than a process that is continually developing, being built upon, being refined, being lived. As a consequence, the process of nursing, how it is created in response to someone needing care, can be missing from reflective accounts.

Missing nursing – treating nursing as an event rather than as a process

A week or so after washing Kate's hair a colleague gently asked me: 'Sue, you are a well-paid nurse. What was that all about with washing that patient's hair last week? How do you justify using your time like that?' I replied that it was about being a nurse and meeting someone's care needs. It was about modelling the imperative of care to the nurses on the ward and the consequence of that care. It was about giving the patient a taste of what palliative nursing care was about before she went to the specialist unit, a bodily understanding of what to expect, to help her with the transition of care from being well to living with an illness. It was about reminding me of what it is to be a nurse, of the reasons I want to nurse. The challenge framed hair washing as an event that happened in the past and my response did little to contradict this view. Neither did I examine the transformation of nursing into an event in my reflective account afterwards, even though I felt disappointed with the adequacy of my response. Rather, I looked for an understanding of this disappointment within the difficulty of articulating palliative care nursing, drawing on what others have said about this (extract from reflective diary, April 2003):

> *Several reasons for the partial articulation have been posed, including the dominance of the medical management of symptom*

distress (Aranda, 2001), the hidden, intangible nature of palliative nursing practice (Duke and Copp, 1992) and its conduct in private places, making it invisible (Aranda, 2001) and difficult to justify (Seymour et al., 2002).

I progressed my exploration of the difficulty of articulating palliative care nursing by undertaking a careful analysis of published research. The account is too long to reproduce here, but an extract will illustrate what I am trying to argue (extract from reflective diary, April 2003):

Palliative care nursing provides companionship that mitigates isolation and helplessness felt by patients and family members (Dunne and Sullivan, 2000). This companionship provides support (Raynes, 2000; McCloughlin, 2002; Mok and Chui, 2004; Skilbeck and Seymour, 2002; Wilkes et al., 2000), involving putting people at ease (McCloughlin, 2002), talking, listening, giving information and advice (Skilbeck and Seymour, 2002; Mok and Chui, 2004), and enabling access to resources such as equipment and finances (Wilkes et al., 2000). Nurses also have an important role in explaining illness and treatment and symptom management (Mok and Chui, 2004) and in putting things across in an understandable and easy way (McCloughlin, 2002). When this care is not available, family members feel unsupported (Dunne and Sullivan, 2000).

This extract from my reflective diary shows how my reflection became a theoretical account that transformed nursing to 'things that palliative care nurses do'.

Subverting nursing – the dangers of academic form and rhetoric of evidence-based practice

There are two things that strike me about the theoretical account that resulted from my reflection, the form in which this was expressed and the search for research knowledge that it provoked.

The form in which practice is expressed

When written, such as when required as an academic assessment, reflection can be constrained by the rules of what has been called academic or scientific form. Several authors argue that this form sanitises the emotional and sensuous nature of experience by changing the architecture of the words used to express experience (Leggo 1999; Gadow 2000; Sparkes 2000). An example from my story of caring for Kate illustrates this point: '*Throughout the assessment Kate kept her hand over her head* _as though she was_ trying to hide her hair'. The phrase 'as though she was' suggests that I do not know for sure that this is what Kate was doing, that I am making a suggestion. Yet I do know that Kate was trying to hide her hair. I witnessed her hand coming up to her head as she apologised to the consultant for the state of her hair. I talked to her after the consultant had left to check how she felt about the conversation about hospice admission. I had commented that I had heard what she had said about her hair. Kate told me she was ashamed of her hair and disturbed that the consultant had seen her with it in its current state and that she had been trying to cover as much of it up as possible. Trying to express my experience in academic form has made something that I was sure about into something hesitant.

Another difficulty with academic form is that it is not able to 'tell' experience because it depends on abstracting experience from the time and space in which it occurred (Richardson 1995). The detail of nursing, of washing Kate's hair without exacerbating dizziness or provoking vomiting, and of doing this in bed, in the middle of a busy ward without disrupting the flow of work, is omitted, because one of the rules of academic form is to avoid lengthy description, yet it is this that would tell how something happened. Time and space and the detail transmitted by attending to them provide understanding of the meaning of the experience (Richardson 1995). Bourdieu, a French philosopher, summarises this point well and powerfully. He says that, '. . . science has a time that is not that of practice'; '. . . practice is annihilated when the temporal structure, direction and rhythm _constitutive_ of practice . . .' are removed (Bourdieu 1977, p.9, original emphasis).

Evidence-based practice

The decision to examine published research of palliative care nursing in my reflection of my colleague's challenging question points to another influence in reducing nursing practice to an event or an intervention – policy interpretations of evidence-based practice (EBP). Despite the intended meaning of EBP being the integration of research with judicious clinical judgement (Sackett _et al._ 1996), by concentrating on what works rather than how something works (Clegg 2005), government policy has disconnected practice from research (Bonner 2003). As a consequence, individual nursing expertise is underplayed (Avis and Freshwater 2006).

The interpretation of EBP as research evidence has been a persistent source of the tension accompanying my experience as a reflective practitioner. The research emphasis has influenced my search for theoretical and research explanations of my experience, to validate them through existing empirical evidence, rather than analysing my accounts for the practice theory that is inherently present. As a consequence, in my reflective accounts I subvert my practice experience as a source of knowledge in favour of published knowledge and subvert my right to voice and portray this knowledge. This contradicts my understanding that my nursing knowledge is as important as published knowledge and how I try to protect this source of knowledge in my clinical decision making. Thus in my written reflection on the response I gave to the colleague who asked me about washing Kate's hair I looked to theoretical explanations. In practice, at the time of the challenge, I tried to broaden discussion of what was happening beyond hair-washing, to examples of what nursing is concerned about – meeting care needs, modelling care priorities and the consequences of care to other nurses, facilitating transition of care.

The relationship between research and practice knowledge is explored by Rolfe (2005, p.79). He argues that EBP can be considered a meta-narrative that 'sets the rules for judging the validity of what counts as evidence' or as telling 'the story of how to tell stories'. Meta-narratives are set in opposition to 'little narratives' which tell other stories of the world (Lyotard 1984, cited by Rolfe 2005). Thus, because research is set in opposition to practice (practice as a little narrative), practice-generated knowledge is perceived as 'transgressive' (Fox 2003) since it positions practitioners as creators of knowledge rather than as receivers of knowledge (Gunter 2004).

Reflecting nursing – examining my reflective voice

Fox's (2003) phrase that practice-generated knowledge is transgressive both rings true and troubles me. It rings true with respect to being about what is privileged as valid knowledge. It captures the feeling of difficulty that I experience, akin to swimming across a current (to use Freshwater's (2000) expression), when I articulate my knowledge and offer this in justifying my care decisions in preference to research knowledge. It troubles me in that I recognise within it something about myself and the ways in which I have developed as a reflective practitioner – what I have let happen in my attempts to be reflective.

Griffiths (1998) gives three meanings of voice that are helpful in describing what it is about Fox's (2003) use of transgressive that troubles me. The use of reflection to further my quest to articulate palliative care nursing captures the first of Griffith's meanings of voice: voice as being ascribed to ' . . . "the unheard" in terms of ideas, perspectives' (p.126) – I felt my experience as a palliative care nurse was unheard. However, as I have illustrated, many of my attempts to have voice through reflection have either rendered nursing knowledge as missing or reduced its significance by portraying it as an event or something that can be done rather than something that is created in response to the person for whom I am caring. In short, my attempts to analyse my practice have used something (EBP) that has been developed to assert others' voices (e.g. government policy). Combined with my quest to articulate nursing, my voice has become wrapped up in a power struggle between policy and practice and between palliative medicine and palliative nursing. It is this that disturbs me. This is Griffith's second meaning of voice: 'the relation of voice to power, in terms of agency' (p.126).

In defining her third meaning of voice, Griffiths (1998, p.126) says that it can be thought about in terms of:

> 'underlying metaphors of form or substance: . . . voice can be thought of in terms of air-time or volume in a competitive struggle to get a hearing; or it may be conceptualised as creative and pro-ductive, developing a greater richness of sound, with new themes and harmonies interwoven in the old'.

This meaning of voice captures the two choices I had in continuing my quest to articulate palliative care nursing. I could continue in the way that I had been and recognise and manage the competitive struggle inherent in this approach or I could find another way, one that uses other ways of depicting knowledge. I chose the second, but before it was possible I needed to look more closely at why I was disturbed by the power relation within the second meaning of voice and within Fox's (2003) notion of transgression.

Reflection is about using practice experience for learning and profes-sional development. When I reflect I have a focus that is on my practice and on my learning and I therefore privilege my voice. Other voices are present through the interactions I have with different people (patients, their family members and colleagues), but their voices are re-presented through my voice. I try to avoid the danger of misusing these interactions or of misrepresenting the nature of the interactions (Skeggs 2002) by carefully recording, analysing and portraying the experience in a way that respects the original intent of the interaction.

However, my perceptions about the nature and intention of interac-tions are shaped by the roles and obligations embedded within health-care practice. This informs who has a voice, with respect to how to act, who to relate to and how to relate. It influences my identity as a nurse and my enactment of moral agency (Doane 2002). As Oberle and Hughes (2001) observe, the contextual forces in health care devolve moral agency to medicine; nurses' experience of ethical decision making is of enacting decisions made by others. As much as I would like it not to be the case, I have been socialised to put medical voices before my own, to show respect to medical colleagues and not to be the cause of confrontation or disagreement (Keddy et al. 1996). I have also been socialised to provide selfless care, to put patient and family members' needs before my own (Freshwater 2000), or at least to privilege the patient's voice rather than my own.

It is these health-care norms that explain why I am troubled by the power struggle within having a voice and in Fox's (2003) notion of trans-gression. When I thought more carefully about how I was going to respond differently and depict my practice, I became deeply concerned about expressing my voice over and above patient and colleague voices. I was shocked and distressed to find that my ability to express my voice was still influenced by how I had been socialised. This was so deeply entrenched within me that for some while I was unable to engage in reflection.

Portraying nursing – redefining my reflective voice

The experimenting with different narrative forms that I described in the last edition of this book helped me to begin to reflect again (Duke 2000). Having a new role as a nurse consultant often meant that I did not know why something was troubling me. Media such as poetry and collage helped me to understand what to focus on in order that I could begin the reflective process in my attempts to understand my practice and the influencing issues. Sometimes these forms also enabled me to express my experience when it otherwise felt contrary to my socialisation. For example, the poem 'Vampires, pirates and aliens' that I included in the last edition of this book tells the experience of finding my place as a nurse consultant in an acute hospital and the response of other col-leagues to this role (Duke 2004, pp.152–153). Shaping this experience by using analogies helped me to depict the experience without it being critical of any particular person or discipline.

> Vampires suck my blood
> And wait for me to turn
> Like them, competitive.
> I strive to stay alive,
> And resist the fanged club
> Instead, collaborate.
>
> Pirates treat me as role
> Contender, trespasser,
> Accuse me of plunder.
> I am no skills thief, but
> See red Jolly Rogers
> Warning, Hold no quarter!
>
> Aliens baffle me
> Their culture quite unique.
> We find no meeting space
> In which to hold debate,
> Tentatively touch it,
> Learn to communicate.

The sociologists
Tell me that these three villains
Have other names instead.
Tell how professionals
Keep strangers out, double
Closure I read about.

The dangers of these foes
Include demarcation
and peer separation,
Designed to increase power
And increase influence,
Instead makes enemies.

Vampires, pirates, aliens
Symbolic experience.
Remind me to value
the nurse in consultancy.
Warns me not to oppress
Others or indoctrinate.

This experimentation with differing forms of expression has also been the way in which I have redefined my reflective voice. It has enabled me to evaluate my role as a nurse consultant and find a more adequate voice in which to express my expertise. In finding this voice I have combined reflective documentation of my day-to-day practice with narrative and reflective analysis of this experience. In narrative analysis, the relationship between analysis and knowledge is considered to be embedded within the narrative. The narrative is seen as both the receptacle for knowing and the means by which knowing can be constructed and communicated. The process of analysis seeks to reveal possible ways of knowing the experience narrated rather than judging the adequacy of practice. This has helped me to avoid immediately turning to empirical evidence for justification and validation.

There is no one approach to narrative analysis (Cortazzi 1993; Reissman 1993; Lieblich *et al.* 1998). Approaches vary according to discipline focus (Cortazzi 1993), analytical purpose (Reissman 1993) and narrative focus (Lieblich *et al.* 1998). I found that by attending to the features of narratives, I have been able to draw out aspects of my experience that I have not documented in the first draft of my reflection. These features include identifying storylines and plot lines, examining the stylistic and linguistic features that I use to express my experience, considering what is missing and why, as well as what is included, considering why I chose to reflect upon particular experiences and not others and so forth.

To illustrate how I have integrated these reflective and narrative analyses, and how this has helped me to convey the knowledge inherent in my practice, the next section of the chapter reworks my story of caring for Kate, depicted at the beginning of the chapter. To do this I have used a modified version of Gee's (1991) method of narrative analysis, designed by Crepeau (2000) and the process of reflection described by Duke and Appleton (2000), constructed from a review of the reflection literature.

The analytical process I followed is illustrated in Box 8.1. The first stage of analysis involved organising the reflective account into idea units. An idea unit is a phrase that contains a single piece of new information, frequently distinguished by a pause or change in intonation – 'Kate is a 67-year-old woman' is an example of an idea unit. I divide the text up into idea units by putting a line break at the end of each unit. The text is then 'tidied up' by deleting asides and redundant conjunctives. The next phase involves organising the idea units into stanzas. Some authors do this by reorganising the order of phrases, juxtaposing those with similar themes to form a stanza (Glesne 1997; Carr 2003). I keep the order of the original prose, finding that the inherent structure of reflection provides an internal structure that determines the stanzas. I insert a line break when the focus of the idea units changes. I then label the stanza with the idea expressed in that group of idea units, as exemplified by italics in Box 8.1. The format of the reflection at this stage becomes what some authors have called 'found poetry' (for example, see Richardson 1995).

The next stage is to identify the basic plot structure of the narrative. To do this I use Labov and Waletzky's (1967) analytical scheme. This scheme has a six-part structure that identifies the temporal ordering of events (Mishler 1986). Cortazzi (1993, p.45) describes the features of this scheme as answers to audience questions:

Abstract	What was this about?
Orientation	Who? When? What? Where?
Complication	Then what happened?
Evaluation	So what?
Result	What finally happened?
Coda	Close

A structural analysis can depict the nature of experience for the narrator – what was focused upon in relation to time (what was valued by being prioritised, for example) and what meanings and values were constructed about the experience (the moral of the story). This analysis of Kate's story identified that there are three storylines in my reflection (labelled 'complicating actions' in Box 8.1): the impact of Kate's symptoms on her independence, Kate's ongoing care plan and Kate's concern about her hair. Any of these storylines could be taken as the focus for critical reflection. I have used the third storyline, Kate's concern about her hair, to take me forward into the reflective stage of analysis, since this prompted

Box 8.1   Structural narrative analysis of caring for Kate

Abstract

Introducing Kate

Kate was a 67-year-old woman
with a brain tumour.
She had been referred to me
for symptom management
and ongoing care planning.

Orientation

Kate's symptoms

She was experiencing dizziness on movement
and associated vomiting
and had a left leg weakness.

Complicating action 1

The impact of Kate's symptoms on her independence

This challenged
her ability to be independent
and influenced her ability to sleep.

Kate's previous independence

Up until recently
Kate had had a part-time job
and helped to care for two grandchildren.

Evaluation 1

The result of referral, of my care on Kate's symptoms

Over the time that I had been seeing her
we had managed to minimise her symptoms.

Contd.

Complicating action 2

Kate's ongoing care plans

Although Kate really wanted to get home
as soon as possible,
we had discussed the possibility
of a hospice admission for rehabilitation.

Evaluation 2

The need for independence

Although initially reluctant
Kate had agreed
that it would be better
to go home more independent
than go home and struggle.

Referral to palliative medicine – progressing ongoing care plan

I asked the palliative medicine consultant
to see Kate
with the view of offering her a bed.

Complicating action 3

Kate's concern about her hair

When I introduced her to the consultant
Kate put her hand up to her head
and said to the consultant,
'Please excuse my hair;
it has not been done for a while.
I usually have it done each week.
I expect it looks a mess'.

The consultant's response to Kate's concern about her hair

The consultant assured her it was fine
and moved on in her assessment
to explore Kate's symptoms
and how she felt about coming to the hospice.

Contd.

Kate's response to the consultant

Throughout the assessment
Kate kept her hand over her hair
as though she was trying to hide her hair.

Evaluation 3

My response: recognising Kate's concern about her hair

I stayed with Kate
after the consultant had gone
and asked her
if she would like me to wash her hair.

Kate's concern about hair washing

Kate explained
that she would be too dizzy having this done
and would be likely to vomit again.

Negotiating what was possible

I said that we could do this for her in bed
and that she would not need to do anything
other than lay flat.
She gave me a very steady look,
smiled and agreed.

Result/coda

Consequences of our care

I went to find a colleague to help me
and after about 30 minutes
we had washed and dried Kate's hair,
given her a blanket bath
and changed her sheets
and she was fast asleep.

my offer to wash her hair and was the source of my colleague's challenge.

The reflective stage of analysis involves asking critical reflective questions of the text in order to understand what is of importance (Box 8.2).

Box 8.2   Reflective analysis

Process identified from literature review	Caring for Kate – reworked reflection
Describe the situation Return and re-tell the experience – significant because it raises awareness of something that does not fit or of unfinished business or because of the feeling evoked.	Kate was a person referred to me from an oncology consultant for symptom management and ongoing care planning. I had minimised her symptoms and after some discussion we had agreed that a period of rehabilitation in a hospice would enable her to regain some independence before being discharged home. I referred Kate to the palliative medicine consultant for assessment for admission. When the consultant introduced herself, Kate put her hand to her head and apologised for the state of her hair: 'Please excuse my hair; it has not been done for a while. I usually have it done each week. I expect it looks a mess'.
Identify a focus Identify what is salient from the incident, what is at the 'heart of the matter'.	The consultant assured her it looked fine and moved on in her assessment to explore Kate's symptoms and how she felt about coming to the hospice. Throughout the assessment Kate kept her hand to her head, hiding her hair.
Analyse your feelings Attend to positive and negative feelings, concerns and thoughts.	1. I was shocked that the palliative medicine consultant had dismissed Kate's concern about her hair. I had seen it as a cue to how she felt (a mismatch between her current self-image and how she would like to present herself). To me, this statement was an opportunity to explore the impact of illness on Kate's identity and the reasons that Kate wanted to come to the hospice – her goals, to be independent. 2. I felt let down and disappointed professionally by my colleague and was angry that this had happened. I had spent a long while talking with Kate about the options for her ongoing care and addressing the pros and cons of these. Kate was worried about going to the hospice and we had needed to work through these worries – concern that by mentioning a hospice as an option I thought that she would not get home, would die

Contd.

Chapter 8

Process identified from literature review	Caring for Kate – reworked reflection
	soon, concern about whether rehabilitation was possible there, concern about being in an environment with older and dying people. The consultant's primary focus on symptom management undermined this work as it did not address Kate's primary reason for requesting admission – to regain some independence. I was also angry because I had spent some time talking to the consultant before she had seen Kate about her goals and reasons for requesting admission. I felt that the work that I had done with Kate had been disrespected.
	3. I was anxious about how Kate felt to have her concern dismissed.
Analyse event/incident with respect to sources of knowledge Integrate knowledge and intuitive and rational thinking as well as personal and ethical knowledge. Scrutinise accuracy of assumptions and test outcomes of previous reflection. Make personal theory public.	*My thinking at the time:* I stayed with Kate after the consultant had gone, although I was torn between this and going with the consultant to talk to her about the conversation and how I felt.
	Testing assumptions: staying with Kate enabled me to know how she felt before talking to the consultant. I also thought that it was important to act with respect to any concerns raised by the consultation as near to the event as possible, otherwise it would look as though I had dismissed Kate's concerns too. I would have the opportunity to talk to the consultant at another time.
	Practice theory: the transition to hospice care can be a difficult one, as it challenges a person's identity in terms of his or her perception of his/her health. It can be related to the stigma around dying that further influences identity. Support facilitates this transition and contributes to achieving the potential of hospice care.
	Summary of research knowledge: Skilbeck and Payne (2005, p.329) commented, '. . . although patients use the language of symptoms and problems, they do not simply focus on disease status. Rather they attach personal meaning to

Contd.

Process identified from literature review	Caring for Kate – reworked reflection

their illness experiences and their problems. When individual meanings are not considered there is a danger that care becomes directed at the problem, rather than at the person experiencing the problem, and this is depersonalising for them'.

Analyse contextual factors influencing situation
Described as the 'where in' factors of nursing – professional responsibilities and boundaries of role, barriers that constrain nurses' therapeutic potential, ethics related to the situation, the moral relationship between practice and action, whose voice is heard and the organisational constraints embedded within the incident, such as funding and policy issues.

Professional responsibilities and boundaries of role: I have a responsibility to Kate, to the ward medical and nursing team caring for Kate, to the hospital palliative care team (where I am based), to the oncologist who referred Kate to me and to the organisation that employs me. I have professional responsibilities to the palliative medicine consultant with respect to appropriate referral of people with specialist palliative care needs and to ensure effective communication to facilitate referral and transfer of care. I have professional responsibilities to myself to know the limits of my skills and capabilities and to seek advice where my practice is approaching these limits in order to develop my skills and act safely.

Barriers that constrain my therapeutic potential: differing priorities between nursing and medicine; in this instance there was a conflict of priority between the goal of enhancing independence and symptomology. Effectively the consultation became a screening conversation for hospice admission rather than an exploration of Kate's needs and how the hospice service might enable these needs to be met in a timely and skilled way.

Moral relationship between practice and action:

- Moral stance as above in staying with Kate rather than going with the consultant.
- Also a moral relationship between practice and action in my decision to wash Kate's hair rather than asking one of the nurses on the ward to do it. I was confident that if I had asked the ward nurses to wash Kate's hair they would have done so a bit later in

Contd.

Process identified from literature review	Caring for Kate – reworked reflection
	the day. I chose to do this work myself because I wanted it to be connected to the consultation with the consultant. I had a good relationship with ward nurses and had tried to develop this as a partnership of care that occasionally included contributing to delivering care, and so it was both acceptable to them for me to wash Kate's hair and not out of the ordinary in how I work with them as a team. Developing this relationship with them enabled me to have the choice of best action in this situation.
	• The act of hair washing enabled these concerns to be aired and the importance of these to be known – that it was less about not being able to do this for herself so much as how her appearance challenged her sense of self, her hair being an important expression of her self, the importance of weekly hairdresser visits, and hair being an important source of self.
	Whose voice is heard: the consultant's voice was heard. Kate's voice was dismissed and so was my voice (the reasoning I had discussed with the consultant for referral). Washing Kate's hair became a way in which I could reassert both of our voices – what was of importance to Kate and the nursing potential to work with her to achieve this.
	Organisational constraints: the key constraint is the way in which palliative care referrals are actioned – I can make a referral for a hospice admission, but the palliative medicine consultants decide about the appropriateness of referrals and usually want to assess the patient before agreeing to a referral. This feels like a vetting process and brings with it dangers such as the one experienced with Kate. This is more likely to occur when the reason for referral is not predominately a medical one, such as in Kate's case, since medical reasons for admission are given more importance than therapy or nursing reasons.
	Contd.

Process identified from literature review	Caring for Kate – reworked reflection
Synthesise existing knowledge with that learnt as a consequence of this reflection Link experience and theory, reconstitute assumptions to make inclusive and integrative, interpret situation as appropriate.	My assumption that Kate's concerns had been sidestepped was confirmed by her in our conversation after the consultant had left.
Evaluate situation and own learning Raise implications for own practice and learning, decisions about what has been learnt and what is of value in future practice.	This raises a question about why I did not act upon my inclination that this was the case at the time it happened. I reinforced the reasons for requesting admission when the consultant raised the issue of how Kate felt about coming to the hospice but did not bring the consultant back to Kate's comment at that particular time. I think some of this is due to the organisational referrals barriers between the hospital and hospice – because of the 'vetting' process I can feel hostage to the consultant's opinion – of patients' needs for hospice care and of their opinion about my assessment of need – if consultants disagree about my assessment, the request for admission is turned down and this can have consequences for the relationship that I have with patients. As a consequence I act in a way that I think best to achieve the desired outcome and sometimes this means I do not say what I would like to for fear that this will negatively influence the decision. In this way, the referral process can be a place where professional power relations are played out – a place where I can be kept in my place as a nurse consultant.
Action plan Identify the consequent or potential change in practice and in own learning as a result of reflecting on this situation. Consider how this can inform intentional practice, change in practice and change in self. Plan how this will be achieved and carry through.	I talked to the consultant about what had happened in a conversation that was about planning Kate's admission. I tried in future interactions not to act in a way that was about being a hostage to the consultant's decision. I raised the question of the referral process to the hospice in several practice development meetings. I further reflected on the referral process as a 'liminal space' in assessment of patients' needs.

Chapter 8

Retelling the story of caring for Kate

The narrative and reflective analysis has drawn out some new understandings about caring for Kate. The following are not necessarily the only ones that could have been chosen; they are the ones that are striking to me at the time that I write this chapter.

When I originally addressed my colleague's challenge I focused on the role of nursing – what I achieved as a nurse by washing Kate's hair. The analysis has shown me that something else was in play in this situation – my role in referral of patients to hospice care and how this is a space in which interprofessional power relations can be played out and the consequent influence that this has on my practice. I explain this in the evaluation section in Box 8.2 as being held hostage by the process of assessment for hospice admission, that this process can become a vetting process of my skills in assessing patient need. As a consequence I felt let down, disappointed, angry and undermined. The analysis points to interprofessional power relations as determining who has voice in this process. In this situation Kate's voice was dismissed, my voice was undermined and the consultant's voice was privileged.

The analysis also highlights the process of brokering involved in referral, in this case to hospice care. Brokering is about working between teams or organisations. In this case I was acting as a broker for Kate between the consultant oncologist and the palliative medicine consultant. Much of the work of brokering is about aligning expectations, addressing conflicts of interest and mobilising action (Wenger 1998; Duke 2007). The analysis points to how I compensated for the lack of attention to Kate's concern in the consultation with the palliative medicine consultant (Table 8.1). I reconciled this experience with one in which her concerns were addressed, to avert a change of decision about Kate's part regarding hospice admission, because I believed that this was a decision that had the best potential, out of the options available, to achieve Kate's goals.

How has reworking Kate's story contributed to my understanding of my practice?

These two themes of power interrelations in the referral process and brokering this process are present in many of the reflective accounts of my practice. In the evaluation of my role as nurse consultant in palliative care (Duke 2007) I synthesised the analysis of these accounts into a narrative that depicts my experience. Whilst my analysis for caring for Kate was not included in this work (it has been undertaken specifically for this chapter), it 'rings true' with the experiences analysed for the evaluation. Collating experience in this way enables me to portray my practice with

Table 8.1 Brokering access to hospice care for Kate

Process of brokering activity (Wenger 1998; Duke 2007)	How brokering activity relates to visibility–invisibility as a co-existent agency	Caring for Kate
Orientation	To recognise something that was previously invisible. For example: • becoming alerted to a patient who was not comfortable when I thought that he/she was comfortable; • picking up on others' concerns, e.g. how a referral is expressed, how an account of a patient on the caseload is expressed.	When I introduced her to the consultant Kate put her hand up to her head and said to the consultant, 'Please excuse my hair; it has not been done for a while. I usually have it done each week. I expect it looks a mess'.
Align expectations	To make sense of why something has become visible. To understand what has gone before – what was invisible. For example: • through patient assessment process: listening to nurses' narratives of care and patient and family narratives of their experiences of illness; • through the colleague supervision process: listening to their narratives of practice, asking questions to clarify their actions; • through drawing up agreements (e.g. role responsibilities, referral criteria).	The consultant assured her it was fine and moved on in her assessment to explore Kate's symptoms and how she felt about coming to the hospice. Throughout the assessment Kate kept her hand over her hair as though she was trying to hide her hair.

Contd.

Table 8.1   Contd.

Process of brokering activity (Wenger 1998; Duke 2007)	How brokering activity relates to visibility–invisibility as a co-existent agency	Caring for Kate
Address conflicts of interest	To recognise possible aspects of conflict. For example, recognising: • where something has been done or not done that compromises what has been negotiated; • when a practitioner or team is 'over-involved' and in danger of taking over and deskilling another practitioner/team.	I stayed with Kate after the consultant had gone and asked her if she would like me to wash her hair.
Mobilise attention	To negotiate and action a mutually agreed plan – to make expectations explicit/visible. For example: • bringing attention to the issues identified on assessment or through supervision; • discussing how these issues might be addressed; • agreeing an action plan and responsibilities in relation to the plan.	Kate explained that she would be too dizzy having this done and would be likely to vomit again. I said we could do this for her in bed and that she would not need to do anything other than lie flat. She gave me a steady look, smiled and agreed.

Contd.

Table 8.1   Contd.

Process of brokering activity (Wenger 1998; Duke 2007)	How brokering activity relates to visibility–invisibility as a co-existent agency	Caring for Kate
Translation	To make the meaning of something visible. For example: • modelling through nursing the meaning of palliative care; • explaining to the ward team my assessment and how this has influenced the plan I am suggesting, pointing to the knowledge and evidence that I am using to make this plan.	I went to get a colleague to help me and after 30 minutes we had washed and dried Kate's hair, given her a blanket bath and changed her sheets and she was fast asleep.
Co-ordination	To act as a go-between with the teams involved. For example: • discussing with everyone involved what the plan is, explaining how I arrived at this plan, and making expectations for their and my actions explicit; • making referrals to appropriate specialists.	

authority. Here are some extracts of how I have described the power relations in the referral process. The text in italics is taken from my reflective accounts; the text in normal font is taken from the analysis:

My attempts to broker access (to hospice care)
provoked the unfolding of an inter-relation
that became enacted in a powerful dynamic
between negotiated expectations
and impotent frustration.

The balance negotiated
between palliative care nurse and medical consultant
wobbled as the power relations played out. . . .

Sometimes the power relations were played out as if
the medical voice in consultancy had more legitimacy. . . .

Sometimes the power inter-relation
was played out as transgressions.

My transgression was towards
the functions agreed
to be part of palliative medicine –
not intentionally, as in being confrontational
but not unintentionally either.

My transgressive movement
was to do with providing comfort
to the people for whom I was caring.
Rather than expecting patients to wait
for palliative medicine advice,
I instigated care, because I had developed the skill
to induce comfort.

As I transgressed,
the voice of palliative medicine
increased
and tried to equalise the balance
by transgressing into my negotiated spaces,
the struggle over admission decisions indicative of this,
the agreement that I would triage patients for admission
often ignored.

The emotional impact of these power inter-relations:

stifling me
as I try and support the fall-out in the team
and manage my self.

They are paralysing me
from moving forward,
invoking my socialisation as a nurse.
I'm finding it really difficult to quash them
and instead feel like I have no choice
in how I act, other than to conform.

. . . We agreed that I would triage patients for hospice admission
according to their needs.
Yet I was not often involved in admission decisions. . . .

The meaning of palliative care . . .
consultant voice and choice . . .
Whereas
hospital patients
and the hospital nurses
had no voice
and the hospital palliative care team
had choice (to be involved)
but no voice to influence hospice admission.
No voice in decisions
other than to offer information.
The ward and hospital teams
perceived as useful
but not as partners in palliative care.

How has analysing my experience of caring for Kate contributed to understanding how I would respond to my colleague's challenge now?

Analysing my experience of caring for Kate enables me to reconsider
how I would respond to my colleague's challenge, 'What was that all
about with the hair-washing last week, Sue? You are a well-paid nurse.
How can you justify that use of your time?' At the time I justified it in
terms of the assumption that being a well-paid nurse should not mean
that I do not engage in direct care, that there are good reasons why I
should continue to model such care and the consequences of such care,
and that some of these reasons are to do with what it is to be a specialist
in palliative care.

 I would now address the challenge very differently. I would not shy
away from what had happened that resulted in me offering to wash this
person's hair. I would discuss the interaction with the consultant that was
the stem of the offer and how washing Kate's hair was part of the process

of brokering access to hospice care, of reconciling what I had perceived to be the deficiencies of the consultant's assessment and of preparing Kate for a transfer of care. I would discuss the organisational barriers in the referral process as a consequence of how referral was managed and the difficulty of my position as a broker in this process. I would point out the skill I use to manage this position and the things that I am working on to assert my voice and patients' voices in this process. I would emphasise the importance of the relationships that I have developed with the ward nurses that made washing Kate's hair acceptable and the skill inherent in developing these relationships. I would discuss the support that these relationships provide to me in my work by enabling me to consider otherwise 'out of bounds' activities and the importance of participation in nursing care in sustaining me in what is a difficult and challenging role.

Assessing my relationship with reflection in my journey as an experienced practitioner: a means by which I express my moral identity as a nurse

Reflection has been a companion in my journey as an experienced nurse. It is a means through which I assess what is 'right', how I assess the moral quality of my practice and the stance I take as a practitioner within this practice. For example, my analysis of caring for Kate assessed whether it was 'right' that I washed her hair and it also assessed the weight of this moral decision. This moral assessment is also about equity, freedom and justice (Habermas 1972; Carr and Kemmis 1986; Mezirow and Associates 1991), for example, understanding whose voice is privileged and how this is influenced. This enables an understanding of how the social context influences how things are known (Habermas 1972) and enables me to understand how to challenge contextual influences that constrain people's voices and influence their care.

   This chapter describes the contours of my journey with reflection, how I have tried to develop skills in reflection not only to enhance my understanding of my practice but also to develop other people's understanding of nursing practice. I know reflection as being about actively working with my experience, as Boud and colleagues describe (Boud et al. 1993), as well as being about myself, who I am as a whole person, and how this is influenced by the people with whom I work. The first half of the chapter describes how sometimes my attempts to be reflective have suffered from some of the monological dangers described by Bleakley (2000). Rather than being dialogical and relational, between my practice and myself, it was focused on myself in my quest to articulate palliative care nursing, or away from myself in my attempts to justify or validate my experience through the research literature.

The second half of the chapter describes how I have tried to revision my reflective voice to find one that draws from the accounts of my experience. Combining some of the analytical features of narrative has encouraged me to consider how I have depicted myself and why (Frank 2000) and to understand that my accounts of practice are both a receptacle and a source of knowledge. Rather than assuming what the focus of an account might be, narrative analysis processes have helped me identify this focus, and, as with the example of analysing my care of Kate, to find something that I had not appreciated was present. McLoughlin (2003, p.67) has a good way of expressing this as a reminder of not jumping to assumptions in analysis: ' . . . discovery often comes from making use of information previously regarded as useless or unimportant'. I find that the multi-layered approach provided by combining narrative and reflective analysis enables a more inclusive analysis to emerge. It situates the focus within the narrative of practice, rather than outside of it.

By combining the outcomes of analysing many accounts of my practice I have also found a way of evaluating my practice and in this way found a way to voice my experience as a palliative care nurse, in an authoritative yet authentic way. This voice is about my identity as a nurse, the moral standpoint I adopt and through which I practice. In this way, reflection, the process by which I assess the morality of my practice, is closely tied with my identity, the moral stance I adopt as a nurse.

References

Aitchinson, J. and Graham, P. (1989) Potato crisp pedagogy. In: *Experiential Learning in Formal and Non-formal Education* (ed. C. Criticus), pp. 15–21. Media Resource Centre, University of Natal, Durban.

Aranda, S.K. (2001) Silent voices, hidden practices: exploring undiscovered aspects of cancer nursing. *International Journal of Palliative Care*, **7** (4), 178–185.

Avis, M. and Freshwater, D. (2006) Evidence for practice, epistemology and critical reflection. *Nursing Philosophy*, **7**, 216–224.

Bleakley, A. (2000) Writing with invisible ink: narrative, confessionalism and reflective practice. *Reflective Practice*, **1** (1), 11–24.

Bonner, L. (2003) Using theory-based evaluation to build evidence-based health and social care policy and practice. *Critical Public Health*, **13** (1), 77–92.

Boud, D., Cohen, R. and Walker, D. (1993) Understanding learning from experience. In: *Using Learning from Experience* (eds D. Boud, R. Cohen and D. Walker), pp. 1–18. Open University Press, Buckingham.

Bourdieu, P. (1977) *Outline of a Theory of Practice*. Cambridge University Press, Cambridge.

Boyd, E.M. and Fales, A.W. (1983) Reflective learning: key to learning from experience. *Journal of Humanistic Psychology*, **23** (2), 99–117.

Brookfield, S. (1996) On impostership, cultural suicide and other dangers: how nurses learn critical thinking. *Journal of Continuing Education in Nursing*, **24**, 197–205.

Carr, J.M. (2003) Poetic expressions of vigilance. *Qualitative Health Research*, **13** (9), 1324–1331.

Carr, W. and Kemmis, S. (1986) *Becoming Critical: Education, Knowledge and Action Research*. The Falmer Press, London.

Clegg, S. (2005) Evidence-based practice in educational research: a critical realist critique of systematic review. *British Journal of Sociology of Education*, **26** (3), 415–428.

Cortazzi, M. (1993) *Narrative Analysis*. Routledge Falmer, London.

Crepeau, E. (2000) Reconstructing Gloria: a narrative analysis of team meetings. *Qualitative Health Research*, **10** (6), 766–787.

Doane, G.A.H. (2002) Am I still ethical? The socially-mediated process of nurses' moral identity. *Nursing Ethics*, **9** (6), 623–635.

Duke, S. (2000) The experience of becoming reflective. In: *Reflective Practice in Nursing* (eds S. Burns and C. Bulman), 2nd edn, pp. 137–154. Blackwell Publishing, Oxford.

Duke, S. (2004) When reflection becomes a cul-de-sac – strategies to find the focus and move on. In: *Reflective Practice in Nursing* (eds C. Bulman and S. Schutz), 3rd edn, pp. 146–160. Blackwell Publishing, Oxford.

Duke, S. (2007) *A narrative case study evaluation of the role of nurse consultant in palliative care*. PhD thesis, University of Southampton.

Duke, S. and Appleton, J. (2000) The use of reflection in a palliative care programme: a quantitative study of the development of reflective skills over an academic year. *Journal of Advanced Nursing*, **32** (6), 1557–1568.

Duke, S. and Copp, G. (1992) Hidden nursing. *Nursing Times*, **22** (88), 40–42.

Dunne, K. and Sullivan, K. (2000) Family experiences of palliative care in the acute hospital setting. *International Journal of Palliative Nursing*, **6** (4), 170–178.

Fox, N.J. (2003) Practice-based evidence: towards collaborative and transgressive research. *Sociology*, **37** (1), 81–102.

Frank, A. (1995) *The Wounded Storyteller*. University of Chicago Press, Chicago.

Frank, A.W. (2000) The standpoint of the storyteller. *Qualitative Health Research*, **10** (3), 354–365.

Freshwater, D. (2000) Crosscurrents: against cultural narration in nursing. *Journal of Advanced Nursing*, **32** (2), 481–484.

Gadow, S. (2000) Philosophy as falling: aiming for grace. *Nursing Philosophy*, **1**, 89–97.

Gee, J.P. (1991) A linguistic approach to narrative. *Journal of Narrative and Life History*, **1** (1), 15–39.

Glesne, C. (1997) That rare feeling: re-presenting research through poetic transcription. *Qualitative Inquiry*, **3**, 202–221.

Griffiths, M. (1998) *Educational Research for Social Justice*. Open University Press, Buckingham.

Gunter, H. (2004) Labels and labelling in the field of educational leadership. *Discourse: Studies in the Cultural Politics of Education*, **25** (1), 21–41.

Habermas, J. (1972) *Knowledge and Human Interest*, 2nd edn. Heinemann, London.

Keddy, B., Gillis, M.J., Jacobs, P., Burton, H. and Rogers, M. (1996) The doctor–nurse relationship: a historical perspective. *Journal of Advanced Nursing*, **11**, 745–753.

Labov, W. and Waletzky, J. (1967) Narrative analysis: oral versions of personal experience. In: *Essays on the Verbal and Visual Arts* (ed. J. Helm), pp. 12–44. University of Washington Press, Seattle.

Leggo, C. (1999) Research as poetic illumination: twenty-six ways of listening to light. *Journal of Educational Thought*, **33** (2), 113–133.

Lieblich, A., Tuval-Mashiach, R. and Zilber, T. (1998) *Narrative Research*. Sage, Thousand Oaks.

McLoughlin, C. (2003) The feeling of finding out: the role of emotions in research. *Educational Action Research*, **11** (1), 65–77.

McLoughlin, P.A. (2002) Community specialist palliative care: experiences of patients and carers. *International Journal of Palliative Nursing*, **8** (7), 344–353.

Mezirow, J. and Associates (eds) (1991) *Fostering Critical Reflection in Adulthood*. Jossey-Bass, San Francisco.

Mishler, E.G. (1986) *Research Interviewing: Context and Narrative*. Harvard University Press, Cambridge.

Mok, E. and Chiu, P.C. (2004) Nurse–patient relationship in palliative care. *Journal of Advanced Nursing*, **48** (5), 475–483.

Oberle, K. and Hughes, D. (2001) Doctors' and nurses' perceptions of ethical problems in end-of-life decisions. *Journal of Advanced Nursing*, **33** (6), 707–715.

Paley, J. and Eva, G. (2005) Narrative vigilance: the analysis of stories in health care. *Nursing Philosophy*, **6**, 83–97.

Raynes, N.V. (2000) Quality in palliative care services: patients' views. *International Journal of Health Care Quality Assurance*, **13** (3), 106–110.

Reissman, C.K. (1993) *Narrative Analysis*. Sage, London.

Richardson, L. (1995) Narrative and sociology. In: *Representation in Ethnography* (ed. J. Van Mannen), pp. 198–221. Sage, London.

Rolfe, G. (2005) The deconstructing angel: nursing, reflection and evidence-based practice. *Nursing Inquiry*, **12** (2), 78–86.

Sackett, D.L., Rosenberg, W., Gray, J., Haynes, R. and Richardson, W. (1996) Evidence-based medicine: what it is and what it is not. *British Medical Journal*, **312**, 71–72.

Seymour, J., Clark, D., Hughes, P., Bath, P., *et al.* (2002) Clinical nurse specialists in palliative care. Part 3. Issues for the Macmillan nurse role. *Palliative Medicine*, **16**, 386–394.

Skeggs, B. (2002) Techniques for telling the reflexive self. In: *Qualitative Research in Action* (ed. T. May), pp. 349–374. Sage, London.

Skilbeck, J.K. and Payne, S. (2005) End of life care: a discursive analysis of specialist palliative care nursing. *Journal of Advanced Nursing*, **51** (4), 325–334.

Skilbeck, J. and Seymour, J. (2002) Meeting complex needs: an analysis of Macmillan nurses' work with patients. *International Journal of Palliative Nursing*, **8** (12), 574–582.

Sparkes, A.C. (2000) Auto ethnography and narratives of self: reflections on criteria in action. *Sociology of Sports Journal*, **17**, 21–43.

Wenger, E. (1998) *Communities of Practice*. Cambridge University Press, Cambridge.

Wilkes, L., White, K. and O'Riordan, L. (2000) Empowerment through information: supporting rural families of oncology patients in palliative care. *Australian Journal of Rural Health*, **8**, 41–46.

Help to get you started

Chris Bulman

Introduction

So you've decided to 'have a go' at reflection. Perhaps you've been inspired by a colleague, you've been asked to try it out as part of a course or you've been thinking about how you might use it in your personal profile for PREP (Post Education Registration and Practice)? Whatever your reason I believe that critically thinking about your practice, striving to become more self-aware and, where you can, making a commitment to change practice in a positive way, are essential for professional practitioners. It is only through 'having a go' that you can begin to discover what reflection may or may not have to offer you. This might not be apparent straight away; reflection is something that needs to be worked at, and it requires time and commitment to a process that may be painful although one that I believe is worthwhile in the long term. My experience of using reflection and in facilitating its use in students and colleagues tells me that most people are relieved to be offered some words of encouragement as well as some very practical help. There is no doubt in my mind that discourse with others who have some experience of using reflection and being given a few handy hints can boost people's confidence with the whole process. Also artful teachers recognise the need to support students in new ways of thinking and learning about their practice but also realise that critically reflecting on your practice is not an easy journey. Thus here is a final chapter to boost your confidence in 'having a go'.

Why bother to reflect at all?

Wong *et al.* (1997, p.476) made the point that in the real world of practice every nurse–client encounter is unique and there are not always fixed solutions to problems. Consequently they believed that nurses need to review their repertoire of clinical experience and knowledge, before they can suggest innovative ways of 'dealing with complex clinical riddles'.

Jarvis (1992) suggested that reflection is not just thoughtful practice but a learning experience. Just as in life, nursing involves situations that are complex, and if we are to understand nursing and ourselves as people who are nurses, we need to try to make sense of the complexity, as suggested by Heath (1998). The important point here is that this is not just about learning in the traditional academic sense but really is an investment in learning about yourself as a nurse and also incidentally as a person, since you don't stop being a person as soon as you put on a uniform. We bring ourselves to our practice, to every situation that we encounter, however much the traditions of nursing in the past have encouraged us not to do so.

Learning about life and practice

Nursing, as with life in general, is constantly changing, challenging, frustrating and exciting – often all at the same time. Therefore, it is impossible to declare that we have nursing 'in the bag'; that we know all there is to know or that we have reached a final understanding of practice. Consequently in order to continually develop our understanding of practice we require what Dewey (1933) and Eraut (1994) referred to as *intellectual effort* in order to push ourselves further in our inquiry and inquisitiveness about the world. I would prefer to call this *reflective effort*, which incorporates thinking, feeling and action effort, rather than implying that inquiry is only concerned with the propositional. It follows that with reflective effort it is possible that theory development arising from practice can emerge as nurses acquire a more reflective way of practising nursing, giving them the critical insight to 'grow' nursing theory from practice itself.

So it is possible, with some effort, to explore ourselves as individuals and professionals, by reflecting on experiences, in order to develop self-awareness and the ability to self-evaluate. In the last two editions of this book, Sue Duke has written about her journey as a reflective practitioner (Duke 2000, 2004); these chapters are wonderful examples of reflective exploration and development and Sue has continued her journey in this new edition. The reflective approach is typified by growth and learning rather than reliance on ritual and automatic pilot to get us through the day (Schön 1983, 1987; Saylor 1990; Street 1991; Ghaye and Lillyman 1997; Brockbank and McGill 1998; Rolfe *et al.* 2001). This is a key aspect of modern nursing. Indeed, Jarvis (1992) strongly advocated the need for reflective practice since nurses are dealing with people who, because of their individual nature, require them to be responsive and reflective, instead of simply carrying out routine and ritual based on presumption. Reflection also requires a wholehearted approach, as Ghaye and Lillyman (2000, p.97) pointed out:

'It is not something to be "bolted- on" to courses and programmes of study. We do not believe you can profess to be a reflective practitioner for one day a week and some kind of health care worker for the rest. It is not something that you can commodify; just pick up and put down, buy into or not, almost at will.'

Reflective effort and change

In order to be effective in practice there is a requirement to be purposeful and goal directed (Street 1991); thus critical reflection cannot just be concerned with understanding, but must also include locating practice within its social and political structures (Bolton 2005) and in changing practice (Driscoll 2007). In order to achieve this, reflective development needs the right culture, one that is conducive to open inquiry, support and challenge and one based on practice, with theory *related to practice* (Goodman 1984; Mantzoukas and Jasper 2004). This operates on the assumption that people want to strive for change and are not content with their 'lot'. Jarvis and Gibson (1997) commented that, because of Freire's (1972) work, it might be assumed that all reflective learning has to be revolutionary; we should not presume this or that reflective learning will be automatically innovative. It is also interesting to consider whether encouraging individuals to develop reflection is one way to divert the responsibility for practice away from organisations and entirely onto the wonderfully broad shoulders of practitioners.

It is worth noting that action following reflection is not always easy since it takes courage and commitment to fulfill. The outcome of reflection may be about individual effort to change, but it may also mean deciding to take action as a team or organisation. Listening to other practitioners confirms my own experiences that sometimes changing one's own practice may be easier than encouraging a team or organisation to take action. In addition, the freedom to question and challenge is not always present and sometimes circumstances dictate that it is easier to leave well alone than to challenge the status quo. These issues need to be considered, since change may inevitably be slow or even impossible and reflection may result in affirmation of an idea or experience rather than in an immediately perceivable change. Cynicism aside, change and development is possible through reflection, especially where it is supported by colleagues and by the culture that people work within (Smith and Gray 2001; Clouder and Sellars 2004). However, it is always valuable to consider some of the issues in true reflective style!

Another careful word is justified at this point. Although I believe that reflection offers most of us a route toward exploring an ability to be therapeutic in practice, this can only be achieved by fostering self-awareness and an ability to be constructively critical in order to facilitate positive change resulting from reflection. However, this has consequences even though it is worthwhile in the long run, since reflection is not always comfortable; this is a point amply illustrated throughout this book. Critical reflection will mean facing incongruity and uncomfortable facts about yourself, nursing and the health services you work in. You need to consider how you will deal with both the positive and negative aspects before embarking on a reflective pathway. Moreover, educationalists introducing reflection as part of a curriculum need to be aware of this and carefully consider the support required for such an approach (James and Clarke 1994).

Below I summarise the important issues that arise from the discussion above and which I hope you will be able to identify throughout the rest of the book. They are to:

- appreciate that situations in nursing can be complex;
- resolve to try to understand what nursing is about;
- try to be self-aware and to self-evaluate;
- question routine, ritualisation and the 'taken for granted';
- develop and challenge current practice.

Helping you to start

Some of the suggestions mentioned below will seem familiar, as they have been covered in different contexts throughout the book. They are either represented here in a summarised form or developed a little further in order to give you the chance to consider what you need to work on, without needing to plough through the book, except where you may require some further detail. Consequently the following are worth considering:

- working on your skills for reflection;
- using a framework to help you to reflect;
- finding someone to reflect with;
- developing your reflective writing;
- reading some of the literature on reflection;
- having the courage to change and challenge.

A summary of some skills for reflection

Checking out Chapter 2 again would be useful so that you can think about what you need to work on; additionally if you are a teacher it should remind you what you may want to 'stitch in' to your curriculum if you wish to help your students develop these reflective skills. The skills are presented in summarised form below:

- *Self-awareness*: this is about analysis of feelings. It involves an exploration of how a situation has affected you and how you have affected a situation.
- *Description*: the ability to recognise and recollect accurately salient events and key features of an experience and to give a comprehensive, yet concise account of the situation.
- *Critical analysis*: examining the components of a situation, identifying existing knowledge, challenging assumptions and imagining and exploring alternatives. You can use critical analysis of knowledge to weigh up how relevant such knowledge may be to a particular situation you are reflecting on.
- *Synthesis*: the integration of new knowledge with previous knowledge. You can use synthesis in a creative way to solve problems and to predict likely consequences of actions.
- *Evaluation*: evaluation encourages you to make a judgement about the value of something. Synthesis and evaluation are crucial in the development of new perspectives

More help with critical analysis

Critical analysis involves separation of a whole into its component parts and detailed examination of those parts. In order to make judgements about the strengths and weaknesses of the different parts as well as the whole, using a metaphor here may be helpful. For instance, imagine yourself knocking down a brick wall. You stand there, mallet in hand, and gaze at it purposefully. At this stage it is just a pile of bricks in need of demolition. After you've exerted yourself knocking it to the ground, you start to see different things that previously you had not noticed made up the wall – the crumbling mortar that held it together, various very small creatures that had until now made the wall their home, the odd bit of graffiti, the demo' posters that someone had stuck on it. And, of course, the bricks! The point here is that through looking a little closer you can begin to look at the different parts that made up your wall as well as the whole.

The skill of critical analysis is not easy so don't lose heart if you don't get it straight away; use your mentor/supervisor to help you. In summary it involves the following activities:

- identifying existing knowledge relevant to the situation;
- exploring feelings about the situation and the influence of these;
- identifying and challenging assumptions made;
- imagining and exploring other courses of action.

More help with synthesis

- Synthesis involves building up ideas into a connected and coherent whole; it is about original thinking and creativity. (Think about how you would build up a brand new wall!)
- Synthesis in reflective practice involves the integration of new knowledge, feelings or attitudes with previous knowledge, feelings or attitudes; it leads to a fresh insight or new perspective on practice.

Some useful frameworks for reflection

You will find different types of frameworks below that are illustrative of those that qualified and unqualified nurses have used in order to help them with their reflection. They have also been employed by educationalists and researchers alike to qualify reflection. Although you may be filled with enthusiasm to begin to reflect, the dilemma of where to start is common. Consequently, I have found that frameworks help with going about the business of reflection. It may be that you feel comfortable with one particular framework and opt to use it every time you reflect. However, it is not essential to use a framework; some practitioners choose not to.

It is also worth remembering Johns' (2000) caution that frameworks or models are just devices to help you with reflection, they are not designed to impose a prescription of what reflection is. Bolton (2005) made the point that frameworks could be as much about control as guidance and therefore they should be viewed and used with these critiques in mind. Greenwood (1998), critiquing the work of Argyris and Schön (1974), also commented on the lack of 'double loop learning' potential in some of these frameworks, i.e. that they fail to encourage the user to search for alternative actions to achieve the same ends or to examine the appropriateness or propriety of chosen ends; that they do not encourage critical reflection. However, she did overlook the fact that frameworks are not the only thing guiding someone's reflection; the challenge and support of coaching and supervision are an important part of the process. Also whilst some may not overtly promote a critical theory approach, they do at least guide the user to think about critiquing experience for future action and the influences and consequences of action.

The suggestions below are not exhaustive since there are many more available in the literature, but in particular the work of Van Manen (1977), Boud et al. (1985), Ghaye and Lillyman (1997), and Jay and Johnson (2002) all provide help for the reflective practitioner.

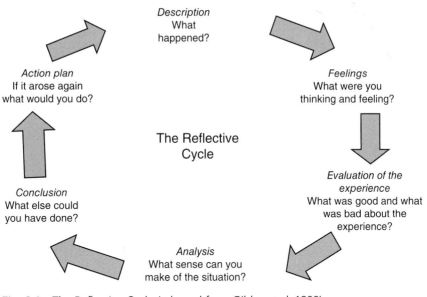

Fig. 9.1   The Reflective Cycle (adapted from Gibbs *et al.* 1988)

The Reflective Cycle (adapted from Gibbs *et al.* 1988) (Fig. 9.1)

When we first started to develop reflective practice at Oxford towards the end of the 1980s we were keen to find a user-friendly framework that would help everyone with the process. At this early stage everyone was a beginner with reflection – teachers and mentors as well as students – so drawing from Gibbs' work on experiential learning proved to be extremely helpful. Graham Gibbs worked at Oxford Polytechnic at the time, so we were able to draw on his expertise and were led to a book on experiential learning he had produced with a project team from the then Birmingham Polytechnic called *Learning by Doing* (Gibbs *et al.* 1988). Several years on, students as well as staff are still finding the so-called Gibbs Cycle adapted from this work of value.

The reflective cycle draws on the work of Kolb (1984) in order to explain how people can learn from their experiences. His work on learning from experience suggested the usefulness of using practice in order to develop and test out theory. This consequently emphasised the importance of drawing on the wealth of experience students inevitably bring to their education and continue to develop over a lifetime. The reflective cycle as used at Oxford was adapted from a cycle of structured debriefing following an experience; this could be from practice, life in general or even from something like a role play. This was recommended as useful since discussions or debriefings can so easily 'lurch from superficial descriptions of what happened to premature conclusions about what to do next, without adequate reflection or analysis' (Gibbs *et al.* 1988, p.46). Gibbs particularly emphasised the requirement to deal with description of both *events* and *feelings* in order to be able to adequately move on to the implications and action plans that arise from an experience reflected on. These were certainly issues that resonated with myself and my colleagues as we have learnt about reflection, used it and facilitated it in others.

- *Description*: What happened? Don't make judgments yet, or try to draw conclusions, simply describe. (N.B. If you are facilitating, hold back from asking questions here; try to allow people to tell their story in their own words.)
- *Feelings*: What were your reactions and feelings? Again, don't move on to analysing these yet.
- *Evaluation*: What was good or bad about the experience? Make value judgments; concentrate on evaluating the way the experience made you feel and react.
- *Analysis*: What sense can you make of the situation? Bring in ideas from outside the experience to help you. What was really going on? Were other people's experiences similar or different to yours? In what ways? What themes, if any, seem to be emerging from your analysis?
- *Conclusions (general)*: What can be concluded, in a general sense, from these experiences and the analysis you have undertaken?
- *Conclusions (specific)*: What can be concluded about your own specific, unique, personal situation or way of working?
- *Personal action plans*: What are you going to do differently in this type of situation next time? What steps are you going to take on the basis of what you have learnt?

Reid (1993) helpfully suggested using the Gibbs Cycle in conjunction with Goodman's (1984) levels of reflection (see below); this is useful in order to challenge yourself to think more critically about the depth of your reflection. Additionally, you do need to accept that the questions in the cycle are pretty broad, so your reflection may not necessarily proceed in a neat cyclical fashion and you will need to reflexively consider *your* effect and influence on practice. Many practitioners like the simplicity of this framework and we have noted over the years that numerous people use it. Through my own recent experiences, I have become uncomfortably aware that I needed to provide more background and detail about the framework in this book in order to help people to get to grips with using it (hence the more detailed inclusions above).

The What? Model of Structured Reflection (Driscoll 2007) (Fig. 9.2; Box 9.1)

John Driscoll is a nurse and teacher and also works as a professional development consultant and coach. Whilst undergoing teacher training,

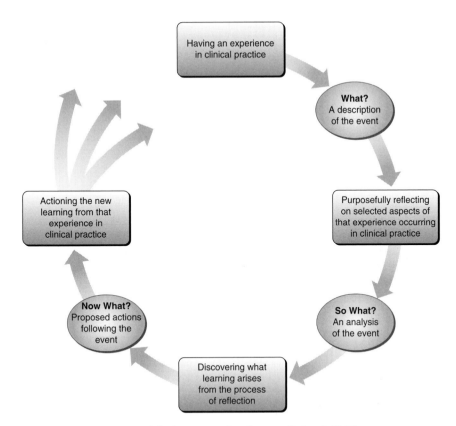

Fig. 9.2   The What? Model of Structured Reflection (Driscoll 2007)

he came up with this model when completing an assignment exploring the use of questioning. Unbeknown to him, Borton (1970) had used similar question headings some years earlier in the USA. Driscoll's model was first published some time ago (Driscoll 1994) and he has developed this latest version which appears below. I think it shows the pragmatic nature of his approach to reflection and is particularly strong on the action element and the requirement to make a difference, influenced by his passion for good coaching.

The Model of Structured Reflection (Chris Johns 2004)

Chris Johns' (2004) model is composed of a series of questions helping the reflective practitioner to tune into an experience and provides organisation and meaning to the process of reflection (Box 9.2). Significantly, the first reflective cue encourages the reflective practitioner to 'bring the mind home'. Johns (2004, p.20) has described this as a 'preparatory cue', placing a person in the 'best position to reflect'. His inspiration here comes from his study of Buddhist meditation, and his 'focus on bringing

Box 9.1 The What? Model of Structured Reflection and associated trigger questions (Driscoll 2007)

1. A description of the event

What? Trigger questions

- What is the purpose of returning to this situation?
- What happened?
- What did I see/do?
- What was my reaction to it?
- What did other people do who were involved in this?

2. An analysis of the event

So What? Trigger questions

- How did I feel at the time of the event?
- Were those feelings I had any different from other people who were also involved at the time?
- Are my feelings now, after the event, any different from what I experienced at the time?
- Do I feel troubled? If so, in what way?
- What were the effects of what I did (or did not do)?
- What positive aspects now emerge for me from the event that happened in practice?
- What have I noticed about my behaviour in practice by taking a more measured look at it?
- What observations does any person helping me to reflect on my practice make of the way I acted at the time?

3. Proposed actions following the event

Now What? Trigger questions

- What are the implications for me and others in clinical practice based on what I have described and analysed?
- What difference does it make if I choose to do nothing?
- WHERE can I get more information to face a similar situation again?
- How could I modify my practice if a similar situation was to happen again?
- What help do I need to help me 'action' the results of my reflections?
- Which aspect should be tackled first?
- How will I notice that I am any different in clinical practice?
- What is the main learning I take from reflecting on my practice in this way?

Box 9.2   Johns' Model of Structured Reflection (Johns and Freshwater 2005, p.3)

Reflective cue	Way of knowing
Bring the mind home	
Focus on a description of an experience that seems significant in some way	Aesthetics
What particular issues seem significant enough to demand attention?	Aesthetics
How were others feeling and what made them feel that way?	Aesthetics
How was I feeling and what made me feel that way?	Personal
What was I trying to achieve, and did I respond effectively?	Aesthetics
What were the consequences of my actions on the patient, others and myself?	Aesthetics
What factors influenced the way I was feeling, thinking or responding?	Personal
What knowledge informed or might have informed me?	Empirics
To what extent did I act for the best and in tune with my values?	Ethics
How does this situation connect with previous experiences?	Reflexivity
How might I respond more effectively given this situation again?	Reflexivity
What would be the consequences of alternative actions for the patient, others and myself?	Reflexivity
How do I *now* feel about this experience?	Reflexivity
Am I more able to support myself and others as a consequence?	Reflexivity
Am I more able to realise desirable practice monitored using appropriate frameworks such as framing perspectives, Carper's fundamental ways of knowing and other maps?	Reflexivity

the mind home helps to shift the balance of seeing reflection as a cognitive activity to a more meditative activity'. Importantly, such a focus requires time, space and an appropriate environment for reflective contemplation. Johns' chapter on 'Becoming Reflective' in Johns (2004, pp.1–44) is useful reading as it is here that he gives more detail and examples regarding the other reflective cues in this model.

Chris Johns developed the model for structured reflection over several years, realising the usefulness of using such a technique, at least in the early stages, to guide people whilst they get going with reflection. The model has emerged through Chris Johns' extensive work through which practitioners have explored their experiences in supervision (for example, Johns 1993, 1994, 1995a, 1995b, 2000, 2004; Johns and Freshwater 2005). His work is extremely well known in nursing and across other disciplines and is certainly worthy of further reading. This version also includes an element of reflexivity, which particularly encourages the experienced practitioner to continue to employ reflective effort in tackling a particular practice issue. This is less evident in other frameworks and is a valuable inclusion.

A reflective framework (Stephenson 1994)

I have included another framework, which poses a series of questions for you to work with (Box 9.3). It emerged from the student experiences of Sarah Stephenson, who wrote in the first edition of this book. Sarah was immersed in reflection throughout her pre-registration, undergraduate studies, and her framework remains worth sharing with others. I have used Stephenson's framework particularly with students reflecting on their clinical experiences and they have found it a useful and challenging guide to reflective tutorial groups and so have I!

Box 9.3   A reflective framework (Stephenson 1994, p.179)

Choose a situation from your placement; ask yourself . . .

- What was my role in this situation?
- Did I feel comfortable or uncomfortable? Why?
- What actions did I take?
- How did I and others act?
- Was it appropriate?
- How could I have improved the situation for myself, the patient, my mentor?
- What can I change in future?
- Do I feel as if I have learnt anything new about myself?
- Did I expect anything different to happen? What and why?
- Has it changed my way of thinking in any way?
- What knowledge from theory and research can I apply to this situation?
- What broader issues, for example ethical, political or social, arise from this situation?
- What do I think about these broader issues?

Frameworks utilising levels of reflection

Theorists have developed work on levels of reflection which have been used by both researchers and educationalists in an attempt to try to qualify people's reflection. They have particular significance in the development of critical reflection and consequently the ability of students to develop and change. A closer look at Mezirow (1981) and Goodman's (1984) work is useful for both nurses and teachers alike in identifying some of the attributes theorists have attached to reflection. They are of course open to the criticism that reflection can be reduced to levels. Yet to the pragmatist, they offer some pointers in determining what the focus of reflection is about.

Mezirow's levels of reflection

Mezirow's (1981) work is influenced by the work of the critical theorist Habermas. Mezirow suggested that adults are capable of being consciously critical or critically reflective and emphasised the importance of self-directed learning. He identified two paths to what he calls perspective transformation or sudden insight into one's assumptions and transitional movement leading to a revision of those assumptions; suggesting that transformation is perhaps the more common of the two. Importantly, Mezirow's work identified the difficulties and problems of consciousness raising that Freire (1972) did not highlight in his work. Mezirow suggested that issues such as difficult negotiation and compromise, stalling, backsliding, self-deception and failure are common features, enough to frighten any enthusiastic teacher or student in their bid to improve reflection! His levels of reflection (Box 9.4), which derived from his collaborative research work on women college returners and their perspective transformations, have captured the interest of both researchers and educationalists in their efforts to find something that helps them to identify reflective capacity in individuals.

Mezirow (1981) saw the first four levels (1–4) as characteristic of what he called consciousness and the last three (5–7) as characteristic of critical consciousness. We do not know how much these are age related, but it is worth remembering that Mezirow studied college returners who were presumably mature women, to begin to develop his critical theory. Importantly, he related critical consciousness and theoretical reflectivity to adult learning, therefore advocating the need to move towards perspective transformation in adult learning. Mezirow viewed perspective transformation as developing an understanding of 'reality' and thus developing a responsibility for decision making, and this he believed was the essence of education. Of course, taking action following perspective transformation is dependent upon the situation and our knowledge and skills as well as our personalities. Mezirow's work therefore makes the point that the

Chapter 9

Box 9.4   Mezirow's levels of reflectivity (adapted from Mezirow 1981)

Mezirow's levels of reflectivity

1. Reflectivity – awareness of a specific perception.
2. Affective reflectivity – awareness of how we feel about the way we are perceiving, thinking or acting and our habits.
3. Discriminant reflectivity – assessment of the efficacy of our perceptions, thoughts, actions and habits of doing things. Identifying immediate courses, recognising reality contexts and identifying our relationships in a situation.
4. Judgemental reflectivity – making/becoming aware of value judgements about perceptions, thoughts, actions and habits.
5. Conceptual reflectivity – self reflection leading to questioning of values.
6. Psychic reflection – recognition of the habit of making precipitant judgements on the basis of limited information. Recognising interests and anticipations influencing our perception, action and thinking.
7. Theoretical reflection – awareness of reasons for our habit of precipitant judgement or conceptual inadequacy. Mezirow (1981) saw this last one as the process central to perspective transformation.

relationship of reflection to change needs to be thoughtfully considered.

Goodman's theory of reflection

Goodman's (1984) theoretical ideas are based on his grounded theory work with student teachers, influenced by the work of Dewey (1933) and Van Manen (1977). Goodman (1984) distinguished three levels of reflection that a reflective practitioner could achieve (Box 9.5). These levels could serve as a broad guide for nurses and for teachers in assessing the quality and depth of reflective work.

   Goodman made the useful point that the focus of reflection needs to be clarified with students; otherwise it is all too easy to end up with most people focusing on the first level of reflection. Whilst such theoretical work is useful in attempting to qualify people's reflection, Goodman himself made the point that reflection is not merely a method of problem solving, but is a way of thinking and being. Goodman made the link that reflection is about the rational (e.g. organisation, selection, judgment and explanation) but also about the intuitive (e.g. imagination, emotions, insight, creativity and empathy). He also drew on Dewey's attitudes

Box 9.5   The focus of reflection (adapted from Goodman 1984)

First level
Reflection to reach given objectives: criteria for reflection are limited to technocratic issues of efficiency, effectiveness and accountability. The worth of objectives is taken for granted; reflection criteria are limited to accountability, efficiency and effectiveness. Students are concerned with what works, and in keeping the status quo.

Second level
Reflection on the relationship between (nursing) principles and practice: there is an assessment of the implications and consequences of actions and beliefs as well as the underlying rationale for practice. A debate over principles and goals can be seen.

Third level
Reflection which besides the above incorporates ethical and political concerns: issues of justice, equality and emancipation enter deliberations over the value of professional goals and practice and the practitioner makes links between the setting of everyday practice and the broader social structure and forces.

required for reflection, namely open-mindedness, responsibility and wholeheartedness. People who are open-minded take a look at the rationale underlying what they initially take for granted as 'right'. They must also be motivated to 'synthesise ideas, make sense out of nonsense and apply information in an inspired direction' (p.20). Finally people need the strength to face insecurities, fears, criticism and upsetting tradition in order to develop change. It is these things, suggested Goodman, that can get in the way of wholeheartedness. Thus courage to analyse and evaluate practice is also necessary.

Summarising a few key messages about frameworks for reflection

My experience tells me that the Reflective Cycle (Gibbs *et al.* 1988) is particularly favoured by many undergraduate students, with the more complex frameworks often being adopted by higher-degree students. The key factor seems to be finding something that helps you to get started and that eventually gives you the confidence to, as Bolton (2001) suggested, deconstruct your own practice. All of the frameworks here have both their strengths and limitations and it is true to say that, once again, more research exploring their use in practice, both clinical and educational, would be welcome. Additionally, frameworks do not encompass all that reflection is or could be; you need to invest in developing the sorts of skills outlined above and think about the influences of coaching and facilitation on reflection and generally have a look at the literature on reflection to get your own critical feel for it.

Finding someone to reflect with

A colleague, mentor or supervisor can provide a sounding board, open up different perspectives and provide support and guidance. It is helpful to find someone who already has experience of using reflection and who is someone that you trust, if you are going to share and explore your experiences and feelings. The coaching and facilitation role cannot be ignored in the reflective process since it is very easy to slip into non-critical, self-affirmation without it. There are those who critique this aspect of reflection as more akin to surveillance and confession (Cotton 2001; Gilbert 2001) and this is provocative reading. Yet it serves to highlight the need to continually critique the development of coaching and facilitation so as not to lose sight of the motivation behind it, which is to *critically explore practice in order to make a positive difference to people in need of nursing*. Take a look at the chapter by Pam Sharp and Charlotte Maddison (Chapter 4) and also by Jane M. Appleton (Chapter 5) to further consider the issues surrounding mentoring and supervision.

Reflective discussion with colleagues is also something that is almost taken for granted or not given the prominence that it deserves. Some people have reflective buddies with whom they regularly discuss their practice. Positive work environments also foster a climate where challenge is expected but supportive discussion is also encouraged. This type of discussion may not be labeled reflection by purists but is part of the process of enquiry in order to move on one's thinking and practice. The key thing is to reflect with people you respect and whose opinion you value and to find an environment where you can be up for a challenge.

Developing your reflective writing

Melanie Jasper's chapter (Chapter 7) offers a wealth of tips and advice on keeping journals for reflective learning. Still, here are a few condensed tips to keep you focused on some of the key issues. Essentially keeping a regular diary is an extremely useful tool, since the memory of events can fade quickly, even for those with the most photographic of memories. You may find it helpful to build up a personal repertoire of experience in your diary, which you will be able to use to reflect back on and draw from as you gain in experience. It is worth setting aside time to write in your diary in a form that feels comfortable to you. Using an attractively bound file or book in which to record your reflections may promote your motivation to write. Johns (1994) suggested splitting each page – using the left-hand side to write up your diary and the right-hand side for further reflections, analysis and notes. He suggested writing down exactly what is said (sentences and key phrases) in order to capture the situation. He also recommended aiming to reflect on both problematic and satisfying experiences. You may wish to record experiences concerning your own patients or situations that seemed dramatic or special in practice. However, it is possible to miss out on seemingly routine or mediocre events which, on reflection, could prove to be useful learning experiences. There is no doubt that diary keeping requires motivation and commitment; some people find it easier to do than others, and other people just don't get along with it. The most important thing is to find a method of contemplating your experiences that works for you.

Educationalists should be aware of the support and guidance needed if diary keeping or journal writing is to be advocated as part of learning about practice. I believe they also need to consider how writing about experience is shared and supported if students are asked to keep journals. The work of Heinrich (1992), Patterson (1995), Richardson and Maltby (1995), Shields (1995), Hargreaves (1997) and Thorpe (2004), amongst others, is worthy of scrutiny before students are exposed to the rigours of diary or journal keeping. (Also see Chapter 5 for further considerations on diary keeping in this area.)

Some practical tips on writing

Writing is something we all have to work at. The tips below are included to help with this effort and were generated from focus group work with some generous-hearted post-registration students who were developing their own reflective writing and didn't mind sharing some of their experiences (Bulman and Burns 2000):

1. Use a reflective framework – stick it on your notice board above your desk where you study; refer to it as you work on your first jottings.
2. Get something down on paper as early as possible, not necessarily something academic or part of assessed work but something you can check out with your mentor in the first instance.
3. Keeping a reflective diary is helpful for some – write down what happened and why, what you learnt and what you would do next time.
4. Look back over your diary – use it to inform the academic work required of you.
5. Make sure you fix up an early meeting with your mentor – and keep it! Check your mentor knows what is expected of you and him or her.

6. Develop a repertoire of practice to draw on and store up experiences that you could use later in your reflective work, by making notes and jotting things down so that important experiences are not lost.
7. Get to know your mentor; use opportunities for reflective conversations.
8. If you can, get to know your tutor; make the most of any individual or group opportunities to get feedback.
9. Write down some reflection, then leave it – go away for a while (about 2 days); you may find it easier to be critical on your return.
10. If you are using a framework, refer to it and ensure all stages are covered in order to complete your analysis.
11. Go deep not wide in your analysis.
12. Live with lack of perfection – realise you won't always achieve the ideal; do what you can with some sense of direction.
13. Seek out colleagues who can and do support you.

Reading exemplars of reflective writing is also valuable to get an idea of how other people have gone about it. You will be able to go back through this book and find some that will be helpful to you, in almost every chapter. For other good and varied exemplars of reflection I would also recommend looking at Rolfe *et al.* (2001), Jasper (2003), Bulman and Schutz (2004), Bolton (2005) and Johns and Freshwater (2005).

Reading the literature

We hope that this book and past editions will provide you with some useful background on reflection. However, in generous academic spirit there are also some others that you will find helpful. These are Johns (2005), Ghaye and Lillyman's books (1997, 2000) and Rolfe *et al.* (2001). Bolton's (2001, 2005) work has particularly caught the imagination of educationalists and Brockbank and McGills' (1998) book is another useful resource for teachers. A critical look at the wealth of discussion articles about reflection in the literature is also worthwhile since it will help to focus you in on the pros and cons surrounding reflection. Here are just a few that span across the last two decades and offer a variety of different views: Clarke (1986), Jarvis (1992), Atkins and Murphy (1993), Day (1993), Greenwood (1993a, 1993b, 1998), Reid (1993), James and Clarke (1994), Richardson (1995), Scanlan and Chernomas (1997), Clinton (1998), Heath (1998), Mallik (1998), Kim (1999), Cotton (2001), Taylor (2003), Clouder and Sellars (2004), and Rolfe and Gardner (2006). Fundamentally, it is helpful to have a wide appreciation of opinions, issues and evidence regarding reflection and consequently to have developed an idea of what you might find helpful in starting to reflect.

Having the courage to change and challenge

My account of a reflective tutorial (below) was prepared for a recent conference paper (Bulman and Schutz 2007). It gives a snapshot of reflecting with student nurses just beginning their pre-registration education. Thinking over such an event from my practice served to reiterate the importance that we should give to listening to and encouraging nurses to get into dialogue about their practice in order to learn from it, right from the start of their education. This process is about supporting and challenging students to develop an *authentic voice*, which truly reflects themselves and their practice:

> *A while ago I was running a reflective tutorial for students who were experiencing their first practice placement. We settled down in a spare room on the ward and I began to ask questions about their first impressions of nursing. One of the students began to talk about starting her degree. As she talked it became apparent that she valued the 'scientific' knowledge that she felt doing a degree was going to give her and the status that this sort of knowledge held. I desperately wanted to challenge this assumption but my experience of facilitating students made me stay quiet and resolve to see how things moved on as we continued with our tutorials over the semester. My decision, by the way, was not as effortless as it seemed since I wasn't sure in that instant whether I was just opting out of the challenge.*
>
> *Several weeks passed and we all sat in another reflective tutorial; again I began by asking the students what had happened to them as they progressively gained some early experiences of nursing. The same student spoke again. She explained that she had become involved in nursing a lady who was dying on the ward; this was her first experience of death. As she gradually helped to care for the patient and her family she described how as a very new student she had to draw on herself as a person and to contemplate how the people that she was caring for were feeling and what she could do that would be helpful to them. Then she recalled her earlier words about the status of the knowledge involved in doing her degree. She went on to explain that she had begun to realise that in this particular situation the so-called scientific knowledge she was describing earlier was not so all-important and that it was learning about herself and how she responded to others in such difficult circumstances that was also worthy and important to her nursing.*
>
> *Through a process of reflecting on her practice and being given space to articulate it I became aware that in only several weeks of*

nursing she had already learnt something important about her knowledge for practice that would stay with her, without me needing to challenge in this case, but simply, with other students, to ask questions and listen. I was glad I had stayed quiet and learnt something valuable myself about challenging students.

I use this example here to illustrate the guts it took for the student above to say that her ideas about nursing knowledge had changed. Such courage is not easy, as discussed earlier, and the current social, political and cultural climate within health care makes this demanding for nurses. You may be fortunate to work in an environment where positive change and constructive challenge are welcomed in the workplace; it is easier then to be brave and voice your reflections on practice (Cullingford 1991). If you are not in such a position you need to seek out supportive and facilitative networks, before you set off on a reflective pathway. Whatever the situation, *contemporary nursing needs nurses who are able to change and challenge*. The organisational structures within practice and education need to work together to facilitate people to do just this; it cannot simply be up to individuals. Otherwise we have to be satisfied with a workforce that does not think too hard about what it does:

> 'Many practitioners locked into a view of themselves as technical experts find nothing in the world of practice to occasion reflection. They have become too skillful at techniques of selective inattention, junk categories and situational control, techniques which they use to preserve the constancy of their knowledge in practice.' (Schön 1983, p.69)

Conclusion

This final chapter offers some condensed assistance in having a go at reflection. It complements and summarises key considerations and critique about reflection presented throughout the book. Reflection has something to offer nurses and I know it is a concept that nurses continue to be interested in. I believe this is much to do with wanting to find ways to articulate professional knowledge to others in order to develop nursing practice, further liberate learning about practice and develop the potency of nursing voices. Ultimately, this motivation is about finding ways to deliver and constructively consider the care given to people in need of nursing. Reflection offers a strategy to do this if it is well supported and challenged by those concerned. It requires educational and clinical organisations to work together.

References

Argyris, C. and Schön, D. (1974) *Theory in Practice.* Jossey Bass, San Francisco.

Atkins, S. and Murphy, C. (1993) Reflection: a review of the literature. *Journal of Advanced Nursing,* **18** (8), 1188–1192.

Bolton, G. (2001) *Reflective Practice. Writing and Professional Development.* Paul Chapman, London.

Bolton, G. (2005). *Reflective Practice: Writing and Professional Development.* Sage, London.

Borton, T. (1970) *Reach, Touch and Teach.* Hutchinson, London.

Boud, D., Keogh, R. and Walker, D. (1985) *Reflection: Turning Learning into Experience.* Kogan Page, London.

Brockbank, A. and McGill, I. (1998) *Facilitating Reflective Learning in Higher Education.* Society for Research into Higher Education/Open University Press, London.

Bulman, C. and Burns, S. (2000) Students' perspectives on reflective practice. In: *Reflective Practice. The Growth of the Professional Practitioner* (eds S. Burns and C. Bulman), 2nd edn. Blackwell Science, Oxford.

Bulman, C. and Schutz, S. (2004) *Reflective Practice in Nursing. The Growth of the Professional Practitioner,* 3rd edn. Blackwell Scientific Publications, Oxford.

Bulman, C. and Schutz, S. (2007) Practical wisdom in professional practice – contemplating some of the issues. Paper presented at the *Creating Phronesis Conference,* June, Aalborg, Denmark.

Clarke, M. (1986) Action and reflection: practice and theory in nursing. *Journal of Advanced Nursing,* **11**, 3–11.

Clinton, M. (1998) On reflection in action: unaddressed issues in re-focusing the debate in reflective practice. *International Journal of Nursing Practice,* **4** (30), 197–203.

Clouder, L. and Sellars, J. (2004) Reflective practice and clinical supervision: an interprofessional perspective. *Journal of Advanced Nursing,* **46** (3), 262–269.

Cotton, A. (2001) Private thoughts in public spheres; issues in reflection and reflective practices in nursing. *Journal of Advanced Nursing,* **36** (4), 512–519.

Cullingford, S. (1991) Learning from experience. *Senior Nurse,* **11** (6), 25–28.

Day, C. (1993) Reflection: a necessary but not sufficient condition for professional development. *British Educational Research Journal,* **19** (1), 83–93.

Dewey, J. (1933) *How We Think. A Restatement of the Relation of Reflective Thinking to the Educative Process.* DC Heath, Massachusetts.

Driscoll, J. (1994) Reflective practice for practice – a framework of structured reflection for clinical areas. *Senior Nurse,* **14** (1), 47–50.

Driscoll, J. (2007) (ed.) *Practising Clinical Supervision: A Reflective Approach for Healthcare Professionals.* Baillière Tindall, Elsevier, Edinburgh, www.supervisionandcoaching.com (accompanying website).

Duke, S. (2000) The experience of becoming reflective. In: *Reflective Practice. The Growth of the Professional Practitioner* (eds S. Burns and C. Bulman), 2nd edn. Blackwell Science, Oxford.

Duke, S. (2004) When reflection becomes a cul-de-sac – strategies to find the focus and move on. In: *Reflective Practice in Nursing. The Growth of the Professional Practitioner* (eds C. Bulman and S. Schutz), 3rd edn. Blackwell Scientific Publications, Oxford.

Eraut, M. (1994) *Developing Professional Knowledge and Competence.* The Falmer Press, London.

Freire, P. (1972) *Pedagogy of the Oppressed.* Herder and Herder, New York.

Ghaye, T. and Lillyman, S. (1997) *Learning Journals and Critical Incidents: Reflective Practice for Health Care Professionals.* Mark Allen Publishing, Dinton.

Ghaye, T. and Lillyman, S. (2000) *Reflection: Principles and Practice for Healthcare Professionals.* Mark Allen Publishing, Dinton.

Gibbs, G., Farmer, B. and Eastcott, D. (1988) *Learning by Doing. A Guide to Teaching and Learning Methods.* FEU, Birmingham Polytechnic.

Gilbert, T. (2001) Reflective practice and clinical supervision: meticulous rituals of the confessional. *Journal of Advanced Nursing*, **36** (2), 199–205.

Goodman, J. (1984) Reflection and teacher education: a case study and theoretical analysis. *Interchange*, **15** (3), 9–26.

Greenwood, J. (1993a) Reflective practice: a critique of the work of Argyris and Schön. *Journal of Advanced Nursing*, **18**, 1183–1187.

Greenwood, J. (1993b) Some considerations concerning practice and feedback in nursing education. *Journal of Advanced Nursing*, **18**, 1999–2002.

Greenwood, J. (1998) The role of reflection in single and double loop learning. *Journal of Advanced Nursing*, **27**, 1048–1053.

Hargreaves, J. (1997) Using patients: exploring the ethical dimension of reflective practice in nurse education. *Journal of Advanced Nursing*, **25**, 223–238.

Heath, H. (1998) Paradigm dialogues and dogma: finding a place for research, nursing models and reflective practice. *Journal of Advanced Nursing*, **28** (2), 288–294.

Heinrich, K.T. (1992) The intimate dialogue: journal writing by students. *Nurse Educator*, **17**, 17–23.

James, C.R. and Clarke, B.A. (1994) Reflective practice in nursing: issues and implications for nursing education. *Nurse Education Today*, **14**, 82–90.

Jarvis, P. (1992) Reflective practice and nursing. *Nurse Education Today*, **12**, 174–181.

Jarvis, P. and Gibson, S. (1997) (eds) *The Teacher, Practitioner and Mentor in Nursing, Midwifery, Health Visiting and the Social Services*, 2nd edn. Stanley Thornes, London.

Jasper, M. (2003) *Beginning Reflective Practice.* Nelson Thornes, Cheltenham.

Jay, J.K. and Johnson, K.L. (2002) Capturing complexity: a typology of reflective practice for teacher education. *Teaching and Teacher Education*, **18**, 73–85.

Johns, C. (1993) Professional supervision. *Journal of Nursing Management*, **1**, 9–18.

Johns, C. (1994) Guided reflection. In: *Reflective Practice in Nursing. The Growth of the Professional Practitioner* (eds A. Palmer, S. Burns and C. Bulman). Blackwell Science, Oxford.

Johns, C. (1995a) The value of reflective practice for nursing. *Journal of Clinical Nursing*, **4**, 23–30.

Johns, C. (1995b) Framing learning through reflection within Carper's fundamental ways of knowing in nursing. *Journal of Advanced Nursing*, **22**, 226–234.

Johns, C. (2000) *Becoming a Reflective Practitioner. A Reflective and Holistic Approach to Clinical Nursing, Practice Development and Clinical Supervision*. Blackwell Science, Oxford.

Johns, C. (2004) *Becoming a Reflective Practitioner*, 2nd edn. Blackwell Publishing, Oxford.

Johns, C. and Freshwater, D. (2005) *Transforming Nursing Through Reflective Practice*, 2nd edn. Blackwell Publishing, Oxford.

Kim, H.S. (1999) Critical reflective inquiry for knowledge development in nursing practice. *Journal of Advanced Nursing*, **29** (50), 1205–1212.

Kolb, D.A. (1984) *Experiential Learning – Experience as the Source of Learning and Development*. Prentice-Hall, New Jersey.

Mallik, M. (1998) The role of nurse educators in the development of reflective practitioners: a selective case study of the Australian and UK experience. *Nurse Education Today*, **18**, 52–63.

Mantzoukas, S. and Jasper, M.A. (2004) Reflective practice and daily ward reality: a covert power game. *Journal of Clinical Nursing*, **13**, 913–924.

Mezirow, J. (1981) A critical theory of adult learning and education. *Adult Education*, **32** (1), 3–24.

Paterson, B.L. (1995) Developing and maintaining reflection in clinical journals. *Nurse Education Today*, **15**, 211–220.

Reid, B. (1993) 'But we're doing it already!' Exploring a response to the concept of reflective practice in order to improve its facilitation. *Nurse Education Today*, **13**, 305–309.

Richardson, G. and Maltby, H. (1995) Reflection on practice: enhancing student learning. *Journal of Advanced Nursing*, **22**, 235–242.

Richardson, R. (1995) Humpty Dumpty: reflection and reflective nursing practice. *Journal of Advanced Nursing*, **21**, 1044–1050.

Rolfe, G. and Gardner, L. (2006) 'Do not ask who I am. . . .' Confession, emancipation and (self)-management through reflection. *Journal of Nursing Management*, **14**, 593–600.

Rolfe, G., Freshwater, D. and Jasper, M. (2001) *Critical Reflection for Nursing and the Helping Professions; a User's Guide*. Palgrave Macmillan, Basingstoke.

Saylor, C.R. (1990) Reflection and professional education: art, science and competency. *Nurse Education*, **15** (2), 8–11.

Scanlan, J.M. and Chernomas, W.M. (1997) Developing the reflective teacher. *Journal of Advanced Nursing*, **25**, 1138–1143.

Schön, D.A. (1983) *The Reflective Practitioner*. Basic Books, Harper Collins, San Francisco.

Schön, D.A. (1987) *Educating the Reflective Practitioner*. Jossey Bass, San Francisco.

Shields, E. (1995) Reflection and learning in student nurses. *Nurse Education Today*, **15**, 452–458.

Smith, P. and Gray, B. (2001) Reassessing the concept of emotional labour in student nurse education: role of link lecturers and mentors in a time of change. *Nurse Education Today*, **21**, 230–237.

Stephenson, S. (1994) Reflection – a student's perspective. In: *Reflective Practice in Nursing. The Growth of the Professional Practitioner* (eds A. Palmer, S. Burns and C. Bulman). Blackwell Science, Oxford.

Street, A. (1991) *From Image to Action: Reflection in Nursing Practice.* Deakin University Press, Geelong.

Taylor, C. (2003) Narrating practice: reflective accounts and the textual construction of reality. *Journal of Advanced Nursing,* **42** (3), 244–251.

Thorpe, K. (2004) Reflective learning journals: from concept to practice. *Reflective Practice,* **5** (3), 327–343.

Van Manen, M. (1977) Linking ways of knowing with ways of being practical. *Curriculum Inquiry,* **6** (3), 205–228.

Wong, F.K.Y., Loke, A.Y.L., Wong, M., Tse, H., Kan, E. and Kember, D. (1997) An action research study into the development of nurses as reflective practitioners. *Journal of Nursing Education,* **36** (10), 476–481.

Index